Brain Candy

Boost Your Brain Power with Vitamins, Supplements, Drugs, and Other Substances

A Comprehensive Guide

Theodore I. Lidsky, Ph.D., and Jay S. Schneider, Ph.D.

A Fireside Book
Published by Simon & Schuster
New York   London   Toronto   Sydney   Singapore

FIRESIDE
Rockefeller Center
1230 Ave of the Americas
New York, NY 10020

Copyright © 2001 by Theodore Lidsky and Jay Schneider

All rights reserved,
including the right of reproduction
in whole or in part in any form.

FIRESIDE and colophon are registered trademarks
of Simon & Schuster, Inc.

For information regarding special discounts for bulk purchases,
please contact Simon & Schuster Special Sales at 1-800-456-6798
or business@simonandschuster.com

Designed by William Ruoto

Manufactured in the United States of America

1   3   5   7   9   10   8   6   4   2

Library of Congress Cataloging-in-Publication Data

Lidsky, Theodore I., 1946–
Brain candy : boost your brain power with vitamins, supplements, drugs, and
other substances : a comprehensive guide / Theodore I. Lidsky and Jay S. Schneider.
p. cm.
Includes index.
1. Nootropic agents.   2. Dietary supplements.   I. Schneider, Jay S., 1956–
II. Title.

RM334.L53 2001
615'.78—dc21   2001032040

ISBN 978-0-684-87080-9   ISBN 0-684-87080-0

This publication contains the opinions and ideas of its authors. It is intended to provide helpful and informative material on the subjects addressed in the publication. It is sold with the understanding that the authors and publisher are not engaged in rendering medical, health, or any other kind of personal professional services in the book. The reader should consult his or her medical, health, or other competent professional before adopting any of the suggestions in this book or drawing inferences from it.

The authors and publisher specifically disclaim all responsibility for any liability, loss, or risk, personal or otherwise, that is incurred as a consequence, directly or indirectly, of the use and application of any of the contents of this book.

To our families, Lorinda and Mercedes Zuck and Diane, Rachel, and Adam Schneider, for their unconditional support of all of our projects

Contents

Introduction 11

1. General Considerations 21
How Do I Know If a Drug Is Worth Taking?

2. "Why Can't I Remember?" 36
The Effects of Biology, Genetics, and Environment
on the Brain

3. Chemistry and the Brain 53
Why Drugs Can Help You Think Better

4. Smart Drugs and Nootropics 68

5. Amino Acids 152

6. Hormones 167

7. Vitamins 186

8.   Oxygen 202

9.   What's in the Research Pipeline? 213

Index 223

Introduction

We got the idea for this book when one of us—Ted Lidsky—developed an aching, arthritic back. As I was unable to get more than partial symptom relief from aspirin, ibuprofen, and acetaminophen, my treating physician suggested an alternative: St. John's Wort. (For reasons that are poorly understood, drugs that are normally prescribed for depression will, if given in very low doses, alleviate certain types of chronic pain.) This herb, now so well known, was unfamiliar to me at that time. My doctor explained that it was a naturally occurring antidepressant that should, like the prescription antidepressants, be effective in treating chronic pain. It was effective; after a few days of taking St. John's Wort, I had better pain relief than I was able to get from ordinary painkillers.

At about the same time as my back pain let up, however, I began to develop a new problem that was even more disconcerting: I began to have increasing trouble speaking. In fact, I had great difficulty thinking of the simple words that were part of my normal vocabulary. My speech repeatedly stalled as I racked my brain to find words that seemed to be right on the tip of my tongue. Since part of my work is public speaking, it was a definite handicap. In searching for the cause of my jumbled words, I stumbled back upon the St. John's Wort, since it was the only recent change I had made in my life. Yet neither the physician who suggested that I use the supplement nor the "authority" in the health food store where I bought it nor the many magazine and journal articles describing St. John's Wort's effects mentioned adverse influences on speech.

Still, I could think of no other explanation, and so as a test, I stopped taking the drug. Miraculously, as my back pain reemerged, so did my ability to find words. I started the St. John's Wort again, my back pain lessened and my speech problems returned. Clearly this was a side effect of the drug that, based on the available information, was impossible to foresee.

Some time after I stopped taking St. John's Wort (for good, this time), I noticed a television commercial for an herb that was touted as being useful in fighting off the effects of aging on memory. Like millions of others in my age bracket, I have noticed a decline in my mental powers as I've grown older. Is it possible that the advertised herb, or any of the other cognitive boosters that are aggressively marketed, actually work? Are they safe? My experience with St. John's Wort, particularly in attempting to get information about its side effects, made me wary. What were, *really*, the benefits and potentially dangerous differences between prescription drugs as compared to the herbs, dietary supplements, and other agents sold in health food stores and other sources of alternative medicines? While it is fairly easy to obtain exhaustive information about the actions and side effects of prescription drugs, it is difficult and often impossible to get similar information about alternative medicines.

I shared my thoughts with my coauthor, Jay Schneider, and together we came up with the concept for this book: to provide unbiased, well-researched information for those people who are considering the benefits and risks of herbs, dietary supplements, or other approaches to improve their mental functioning—brain candy, so to speak.

It is intriguing that despite the questions about alternative medicines, dietary supplements, and herbs, the sale of these products is a multibillion-dollar business. Why, in the face of so many unknowns, are people so willing to buy and take these substances? Since many of us are either baby boomers or the children of baby boomers, perhaps one consequence of our experiences through the sixties and seventies is a tendency to gravitate toward "natural" solutions to our problems. There is not a one of us who hasn't been appalled by the price of prescription drugs. In fact, the more we hear about hospital screwups, misdiagnoses, and harmful treatments doled out by physicians, the less we trust the traditional medical and pharmaceutical establishment to cure our ills and fix our problems. Many of us equate "natural" with "good" whether referring to the food we eat or the drugs we take, yet some of these products may be poisonous or harmful. However, we can't overlook the reality of these herbs finding their way into our daily diet through addition to snack foods and drinks. This movement has so permeated our culture that products such as iced tea spiked with ginkgo and other herbs are common sights on supermarket shelves.

The problem is, our yen for natural remedies to treat our waning mental capacities or prevent their eventual decline can put our overall health at risk. There are many people who will tell you that there is nothing wrong with taking herbs or combinations of herbs to fix your memory or lift you out of a funk. Many of them are sincere and many are not. Some of these advocates either have an equity stake in companies selling these items or, more ethically appalling, sell these products themselves.

The truth is, some remedies available today may cause serious adverse effects such as dangerously increasing blood pressure and altering heart rhythm, life-threatening allergic reactions, kidney and liver failure, and may even be carcinogenic. There is growing evidence that even the most popular remedies out there, St. John's Wort and ginkgo biloba, may have dangerous interactions with various prescription drugs. In fact, the American Society of Anesthesiologists recently issued a warning to consumers using herbal remedies to stop taking them at least two to three weeks before any scheduled surgery due to dangerous and life-threatening interactions of some of these remedies with the drugs used to anesthetize patients during surgery. For example, ginkgo biloba, garlic, ginger, and ginseng may prevent blood clots from forming and lead to excessive blood loss during surgery, while St. John's Wort and kava kava may prolong the sedative effects of anesthesia.

So, who is going to protect us from potentially harming ourselves as we try to find the magic elixir for forgetfulness? Our legislators in Congress? Not likely. In 1994, Congress passed a law, the Dietary Supplement Health and Education Act, that distinguishes between products that claim to "affect the structure or function of the body" and those that claim to prevent, treat, or cure disease. Thus, dietary supplement manufacturers (who have a very effective and powerful lobby in Washington) can market their products without any safety or efficacy testing as required of a pharmaceutical agent, as long they don't make claims related to disease. What about the Food and Drug Administration? This is equally unlikely. The

FDA recently eased restrictions on dietary supplements (herbal remedies are classified as dietary supplements), saying these products can legally claim to treat various symptoms, such as age-related memory loss, that are considered to be common passages of life. This of course was good news for the $6-billion-a-year dietary supplement industry (and personal injury lawyers), but bad news for consumers.

In 1997, the President's Commission on Dietary Supplement Labels recommended that the FDA appoint a committee to evaluate the safety and effectiveness of dietary supplements, but at this time there is no effort under way at the FDA to change the manner in which the agency reviews or regulates homeopathic preparations.

The truth is, the $6 billion worth of dietary supplement pills, capsules, teas, and elixirs used by U.S. consumers each year undergo absolutely no government or industry scrutiny for safety and effectiveness before reaching the store shelves. There are also no manufacturing standards to ensure the quality of the product that you are buying. There is no way for you to know if that bottle of kava kava you just bought really contains what the label says it does and that it is free from harmful contaminants.

If this scares you, it should. It scares us. And that brings us to this book. Dietary supplement manufacturers are going all out to attract consumers who are otherwise healthy individuals who are experiencing normal age-related changes (these often begin in your forties) in their memory and concentration abilities. Forgot the name of the guy you were introduced to a few minutes ago? Forgot where you left your car keys? Middle-age forgetfulness can happen to all of us occasionally and as the population ages (the number of people over age sixty-five will double in the next thirty years), the market for supplements that counteract these cognitive changes will grow. The purpose of this book is to provide you with some objective information about the safety and effectiveness of a wide variety of potentially brain-altering compounds so that you can make educated decisions about whether you want to use them, or not.

Brain Candy is organized into chapters that explain how the effectiveness and risks of drugs are evaluated (Chapter 1), the many environmental and biological factors that affect your ability to remember (Chapter 2), and how the brain stores information (Chapter 3). The remainder of the book discusses the variety of herbs, drugs, and hormones that are either available now (Chapters 4 through 8) or are being investigated in the laboratory (Chapter 9).

Each substance is discussed under the following headings:

What is it? identifies the compound

Its reputation tells you what people claim about the compound

The drug's effect on the brain provides information concerning the biological effects of the substance on the brain

How has it been tested? What are the risks, if any? provides the scientific basis for the claims and lists the risks if these are known

Typical dosages lists the doses of the substance that have been reported as commonly used

Contraindications notes the medical conditions that would render use of the substance dangerous

The plain facts summarizes the information about the compound and, if there is sufficient information on which to base a decision, makes a general recommendation. In addition, to help in the decision-making process we have rated each compound for potential benefits and risks. Benefits are rated on a 6-point scale with 0 being no benefit and 5 considerable benefit. Similarly, risks are also rated on a 6-point scale with 0 indicating no known risk and 5 maximum risk. Risks in the range of 4 or 5 are unacceptable no matter how great the benefits.

Although we have attempted to provide a list of contraindications for the drugs described throughout the book, the following should be noted. Only specific conditions that contraindicate the use of a drug are noted. It should be understood that for each entry, a specific allergy to that drug is a contraindicating condition. Unfortunately, the actions of many of these substances have not been sufficiently documented to enable a comprehensive list of possible risks, adverse reactions, and contraindications. In particular, for example, the effects of the majority of these compounds on pregnancy, the developing fetus, and children have not been studied; therefore, these substances should not be taken when pregnant or be administered to children. Prudence and common sense must be used and a discussion with a competent health professional is strongly recommended before embarking on a course of dietary supplementation.

Ultimately, when it comes to the use of dietary supplements to treat age-related cognitive decline, you need to be an educated but wary consumer. There are some good reference books—for example, the American Pharmaceutical Association's *Practical Guide to Natural Medicines* and the *Physicians' Desk Reference for Herbal Medicines*—that you can go to for information on a wide variety of substances. The Internet can also provide a wealth of information on supplements, medications, and health conditions. A reference book like *The Doctor's Always In*, which we published in 1999, can help you zero in on useful sites and save countless hours of search time. When searching the Internet for medical or drug/supplement information, remember that there is no mechanism in place to monitor Internet health sites or businesses to control for deceptive or false claims and practices. Just because information is easily accessible on the Internet doesn't necessarily mean that the information is good.

Here are some tips for getting the most out of a search for medical, drug, and supplement information on the Internet:

- *Know who's responsible for the site.* Sites posted by government agencies (.gov), universities or other educational institutions (.edu), and reputable organizations (.org) usually contain the most useful and reliable information.
- *Be wary of commercial (.com) sites.* While many commercial sites do provide useful information, be wary of sites that seem to be hyping a product and that provide superficial information in their unabashed attempt to sell you something.
- *Check for the currency of the information and the credentials of the individual(s) posting the information.* Is the information current and up-to-date? Is the information posted by someone with medical or scientific expertise? Are individuals with science or medical expertise consultants or advisors to the site? Are the sources of the information listed, and do they appear to be authoritative?
- *Beware of outlandish claims and testimonials.* Always remember: if a product seems too good to be true, it probably is.

We are not advocating the use of any compounds, nor are we putting a blanket rejection on all dietary supplements. We are merely presenting you with the best and most objective information available on the safety of the various compounds listed and the real scientific evidence (if it exists) to support the use of the supplement. The final decision on whether to use or not use any particular item is yours alone. We hope that you find this book useful.

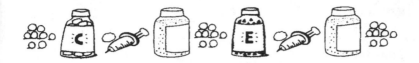

1

General Considerations:
How Do I Know If a Drug Is Worth Taking?

Recently, a colleague of ours complained that he was having difficulty remembering the little things. For example, he had trouble finding his car keys in the morning—he just couldn't remember where he put them. Then he couldn't remember when it was his day to pick the kids up from school. Reluctant to admit he had a problem, he started writing things down. Then he couldn't find the list!

Convinced (by his wife and kids) that he was losing his mind, he went to the local health food store. The clerk guided him to take the supplement choline, because "it contributes to your mental alertness, concentration, and memory." Two weeks later, he was not only forgetting where his keys were, but also whether or not he had taken his choline.

Is it reasonable to presume that something that is advertised and sold as a memory aid will actually improve memory? Maybe yes, maybe no. Since there are few guarantees in life, your wisest bet is to find out, before you take it, what a substance promises and what it delivers—benefits, side effects, and warranties.

Generally, when your doctor prescribes a drug, it's reasonable to believe that the medication will have some predictable and well-known beneficial effect (and often a whole host of side effects). For example, if you have a bacterial infection, the antibiotic drug you are prescribed will have been established to effectively kill bacteria. The drug company that manufactures and sells the drug will package it with an insert that describes not only what conditions this drug is designed to treat, but also how much should be taken, for how long, and the likely side effects you may experience. If you have a regular pharmacist, he or she will check this drug and compare it with any others you're taking to make sure there are no interactions. When you take the drug, there is a strong likelihood that it will treat your infection.

Unfortunately, a product bought in a health food store or ordered over the Internet is not warranted to have the advertised beneficial effect. The reason for this disparity is that prescribed medications are classified as drugs and health food products as dietary supplements. The two are regulated in completely different ways. To understand the vast difference between the classifications and what this means to you, the consumer, let us first discuss exactly what constitutes a drug and what constitutes a dietary supplement.

DRUGS

A drug is defined as a chemical that is used to prevent or treat an illness. Drugs are regulated by the U.S. Food and Drug Administration (FDA) through the Federal Food, Drug, and Cosmetic Act of 1938 and the Kefauver-Harris Drug Amendments of 1962. For all drugs, effectiveness and safety have to be scientifically proven through a systematic process of testing. The testing is first carried out in the laboratory, using animals, to determine whether the drug has an effect on the illness in question and whether the drug is toxic. If the drug has shown possibility in the preclinical testing, then human clinical testing begins.

The Approval Process—Human Testing

Human clinical testing takes place in phases. In Phase One, the drug is given to a small number of healthy people for several months to establish basic information about how it works in people. A primary goal is to see if it is safe, find the most common side effects, and the maximum doses people can take without adverse effects. Data are also gathered to determine the best route of administration (e.g., injection, tablet, patch), what happens to the drug in the body (how well it is absorbed, what organs are affected, how long it stays in the body, and how well it's broken down), and what factors may influence the drug's actions (for example, if men and women react differently or if food or drink affect the drug's properties).

If no major problems are detected, the drug moves up to Phase Two testing. In Phase Two, the drug is given to several hundred ill patients for up to two years. Researchers test for safety and effectiveness, and closely monitor the effect of the drug on the patients. If it appears to be effective and safe, it enters Phase Three testing. In this stage, the drug is given to up to several thousand ill patients at many different trial sites for one to four years to further test safety and effectiveness and to determine dosage.

As you can see, the approval process for drugs takes an average of eight and one-half years. For every hundred drugs that start in Phase One, less than twenty will pass Phase Three and finally be marketed to the public. The average cost to develop a single drug is $359 million.

What Happens After a Drug Is Approved?

Side effects continue to be monitored after a drug is put on the market through a voluntary reporting program for health professionals called MedWatch. Between June 1993 and July 1994, there were 9,879 reports of adverse drug effects and 1,406 complaints of drug quality. According to David A. Kessler, the former FDA Commissioner, "There is simply no way that we can anticipate all possible effects of a drug or device during the clinical trials that precede approval. A new drug application, for example, typically includes safety data on several hundred to several thousand patients. If an adverse event occurs in one in five thousand, or even one in one thousand users, it could be missed in clinical trials. But it could pose a serious safety problem when the drug is used by many times that number of patients."

These comments have proved to be a vital tool for regulating approved drugs. For example, Felbatol, an antiepileptic drug, was withdrawn from the market by the FDA because this medication caused a rare and potentially fatal blood disease called aplastic anemia in ten patients. It was not seen at all during preapproval testing. Yet, since Felbatol's approval, the rate of aplastic anemia cases in patients taking this drug appears to be about fifty times higher than was expected.

DIETARY SUPPLEMENTS

A dietary (or nutritional) supplement is defined as a product other than tobacco that is intended to supplement the diet, and which contains at least one of the following substances: a vitamin, a mineral, an herb, or an amino acid. Supplements come in a variety of forms, including pills, capsules, tablets, tea, and liquid form and are clearly labeled as "dietary supplement," and it is strictly prohibited to make advertisements or claims on the labeling touting the supplement as a treatment for a specific illness or disease. There are certain health claims for some dietary supplements that have been authorized by the FDA because the product has been tested and found worthy—and these claims may be included on the label. For example, the claim linking folic acid and reduced risk of neural tube defects during pregnancy is authorized, as is the claim that calcium may reduce the risk of osteoporosis.

Health claims that are offered on behalf of dietary supplements are regulated by the Dietary Supplement Health and Education Act (DSHEA) of 1994. The act states that claims of effectiveness in treating health problems cannot be made directly. However, third-party material, if it is in the form of testimonials by users about the product's health benefits, is allowed. The DSHEA maintains that it is the manufacturer's responsibility to ensure that the dietary supplement is safe.

Are Drugs Really Different from Dietary Supplements?

In terms of their effect on the body, there is no difference between a drug and a dietary supplement. Both are chemicals that influence the functioning of the body. Some physicians and drug company executives have argued that drugs are safer than dietary supplements because they are subjected to rigorous testing according to FDA guidelines. But, with all the safety precautions taken for FDA approved drugs, there are still significant dangers. It is estimated that in 1994 alone, prescription drugs caused 106,000 deaths and serious side effects in 2.2 million hospital patients. Dietary supplements are not free from dangers either. The fact that a substance is "natural" or comes from a plant does not automatically guarantee safety. For example, arsenic can be found in the pits of apricots and some grapes, while morphine is derived from the opium poppy. The absence of standardized procedures for evaluating and reporting adverse effects of dietary supplements does not mean that such effects do not exist. Rather, you simply have no easy way find out if there are adverse effects and what these might be.

We can say with certainty that statements concerning the effectiveness of dietary supplements are not always based on as solid scientific grounds as drugs controlled by the FDA. On the other hand, the absence of FDA approval does not indicate that there is no scientific evidence for the effectiveness of a dietary supplement or that the dietary supplement doesn't work. Often, the dietary supplement has not been rigorously tested. The cost of testing a drug according to the FDA guidelines is enormous. Since most of the products available in health food stores cannot be patented, a pharmaceutical company would have no interest in testing such a substance. They could not make enough money on it to justify going through the FDA's procedures for approval. Pharmaceutical companies are only interested in developing unique drugs for which they can hold a patent and monopolize the initial market. Therefore, it is possible that certain dietary supplements are effective but will never go through the FDA for approval as a treatment for a disease because there is no financial incentive.

However, many dietary supplements have been tested in various ways. An educated consumer, if allowed access to the existing information about a particular dietary supplement, can evaluate the evidence and decide whether a treatment is likely to be effective and whether or not it is safe. Unfortunately, much of this information is written for trained researchers and uses technical language and concepts that are difficult to understand without a background in science. In addition, this information is not always easy to find since most of it appears in articles that are written in books and journals that are available only in medical school libraries.

So, to make your life easier, we've condensed this information for you.* In the succeeding chapters of this book, you will find much of what you need to determine the safety and effectiveness of the majority of dietary supplements currently available to treat memory. First, however, let's turn our attention to testing, because you can't evaluate a dietary supplement without understanding how it has been tested.

How Drugs and Dietary Supplements Are Tested

Drugs and dietary supplements are tested on animals and/or humans and each method has inherent strengths and weaknesses. By understanding the differences in testing of various substances, you can better determine if you want to take the risk of ingesting a drug or supplement that may or may not improve or enhance your thinking ability.

---

*Both of us are Ph.D. neuroscientists with a combined fifty years of experience in not only reading and critically evaluating scientific literature but also writing a combined total of more than 150 scientific papers.

ANIMAL TESTING

Many drugs and dietary supplements have been tested using laboratory animals. The generic experiment would compare a "control" group, in which animals receive a substance known to be without effect (placebo), with an "experimental" group in which the animals receive the test drug. To illustrate how this method is applied to drugs that could affect thinking power, let's consider a supplement that is supposed to enhance learning ability. Similar methods would be used if the drug were to be tested for effects on other aspects of cognitive functioning such as attention, memory, or executive functioning (see Chapter 2). Animals in the experimental group that receive the supplement in question would be compared to animals in the control group with respect to how well they learn a task such as pressing a bar for a food reward or learning to avoid an electric shock. If the animals receiving the drug learn more quickly, it can sometimes be concluded that the drug improved learning ability. To reach that conclusion the scientist must first rule out alternative effects of the drug, such as beneficial influences on attention or, in tasks motivated by food reward, increases in hunger or, in tasks motivated by shock avoidance, drug-induced increases in fear or pain sensitivity.

A beneficial effect of a drug in an experiment using animals is often the basis for a scientist to investigate the effects of the drug in humans. However, such an effect is not a guarantee that the drug will be of any use to people and, in the absence of compelling evidence concerning the drug's safety and effectiveness in humans, should not be the reason for consumers to try it out on themselves. There are several important reasons to wait for the research to be completed before taking an unknown drug. First, the most obvious, a rat is not a human (despite the sad fact that the reverse is too often the case). Drugs can have different effects in animals than in people. For example, aspirin is usually an effective and relatively safe painkiller in humans but will kill cats. Second, many tasks that are used to test animal learning may not be analogous to the types of things humans do. The majority of experiments testing the effects of dietary supplements use mice or rats in tasks such as solving a maze or avoiding a punishment. Learning that a buzzer warns of an impending electric shock is not the same thing as learning algebra, although it may feel the same for some people.

Although experiments that study the effects of drugs in primates—monkeys and apes—can and do employ behavioral tasks that require cognitive processes that are closely analogous to those of humans, these animals are rarely used to test dietary supplements. As mentioned above, this is largely due to the fact that most of these studies are quite costly and are often underwritten by a third party, generally a pharmaceutical company.

Third, laboratory animal brains are different from human brains. Learning a language, for example, requires a specialized portion of the human brain that has no equivalent in mice or rats. Last, because of the importance of language, humans are very likely to learn tasks in fundamentally different ways than those used by laboratory animals. For example, when a person memorizes the directions for traveling to a new location, he or she is likely to make a mental note of the sequence of left and right turns. A mouse, faced with an analogous task in a maze, will obviously have to use other strategies.

HUMAN TESTING

Testing drugs in people is very similar to testing in laboratory animals. Again, the generic experiment would be to compare a control group with an experimental group to see how quickly they can learn a task. In well-conducted experiments, as with animal studies, people in the control group are treated identically to people in the experimental group, with the exception that the latter receive the test drug while the former are administered a placebo. Any of a variety of cognitive abilities could be tested including concentration, memory, planning, and concept formation. It is critical that the study be double-blind and placebo-controlled.

PLACEBO-CONTROLLED TRIALS

Placebo-controlled means that people in the control group receive a drug known to be ineffective but that, in all other respects, is identical to the test drug. It is important that the control group receive a placebo rather than no drug at all. People who believe they are being treated, even if the treatment is actually without biological effect, will usually do better than people who know they are not being treated. This beneficial result of positive thinking is known as the placebo effect. Sometimes people show a placebo effect merely in response to participating in a study. The positive social experience and camaraderie of sharing similar experiences with others can be very powerful. The enormous power of the placebo effect should not be underestimated, particularly in illnesses in which emotions can play a strong part. "In trials of antidepressants," says Dennis Charney, director of the Yale

Mental Health Clinical Research Center, "it is not uncommon for 65 percent of the patients on the new drug to get better. But 35 percent of the patients in the placebo group also typically improve."* Placebo effects could be considered as treatments for an illness if they could be reliably induced and if they persist. Unfortunately, placebo effects most often do not last indefinitely. Thus, in order for a test drug to be judged as beneficial, it must do better than the effect of positive thinking.

DOUBLE-BLIND AND SINGLE-BLIND

Double-blind means that neither the people who are being tested nor the scientists doing the testing know, during the actual experiment, which people are receiving the test drug and which are receiving the ineffective placebo. To accomplish this, a third party codes the drugs to hide their identity and keeps records to indicate who received which drug. At the completion of testing, the code is broken so that the results can be analyzed. The reason for keeping both the participants in the study and the scientists in the dark is to prevent inadvertent or intentional influencing of the results. Researchers can have preconceived ideas about the effectiveness of a test drug. If they knew who was getting the drug and who was getting the placebo, their biases could influence the way patients were treated in the study and ultimately affect the outcome. In addition, it is often necessary for a drug manufacturer to pay for the testing of one of its own products. The use of double-blind and placebo-controlled

---

*M. Enserink, "Can the Placebo Be the Cure?" *Science* 284: 238, 1999.

studies virtually guarantees objectivity and prevents even the appearance of impropriety or conflict of interest. Double-blind studies are also a good way to measure drug efficacy because the subjects do not know whether they are receiving the test drug or placebo. For example, a subject receiving the test drug might do better if the knowledge of receiving a "memory drug" increased expectations or motivations to learn. Conversely, a participant with the knowledge of receiving the ineffective placebo might be disappointed, less motivated to work, and consequently fare worse while on the drug.

A study in which only the participants are unaware of the type of drug they are receiving is called single-blind. Its results are considered much less persuasive than double-blind studies. Often a single-blind study is done first with a new drug to inform the researchers if there is a high enough likelihood of effectiveness to justify their undertaking the far more involved and costly double-blind trial. While positive results in a single-blind study might be sufficient justification for a scientist to plan future studies, such results are not sufficiently persuasive to justify use by the public at large.

EVALUATING YOUR RISK

Virtually all drugs carry some risk. It's safe to assume that all dietary supplements also carry some risk, although lack of formal regulation means side effects may go unreported. When taking *any* type of product, it is important to weigh the risks against the potential benefits—this is known as the risk/benefit ratio.

Adverse effects of drugs/dietary supplements can be either dramatic and direct or more subtle and indirect. Lobelia, an herb taken as expectorant, antiasthmatic, and antidepressant, manifests direct effects. Taken in high doses, this drug can cause rapid heart rate, coma, and even death. Kava kava, a member of the pepper family taken as a sedative, muscle relaxant, and treatment for anxiety, has both direct and indirect effects. This drug can cause scaly skin rash (direct effect), but more important, when combined with barbiturates (taken for insomnia and epilepsy), can cause overdose with potentially fatal results.

Drug interactions are an important area of medicine that is gaining increasing interest and attention. With prescription drugs, quite a bit is known. For example, combining the anticoagulant Coumadin (frequently prescribed for persons at risk for heart attacks or stroke) with aspirin can lead to fatal hemorrhaging. Similarly, the potentiating effects of alcohol on barbiturates and tranquilizers, though well known, still lead to serious complications and death with disturbing frequency. More recently it has been discovered that grapefruit juice will affect the liver in such a way that certain drugs taken to treat hypertension are not broken down and eliminated from the body as quickly as they should be. Thus, even drinking something as seemingly benign as grapefruit juice can lead to drug overdose.

In contrast to prescription drugs, the study of interactions between dietary supplements and prescription drugs is just beginning and the possibility of interactions with other dietary supplements is largely unexplored. Additionally, adverse effects of drugs sometimes only become apparent after long-term use. There are few if any long-term studies of the effects of dietary supplements.

STANDARDIZATION OF INGREDIENTS

There is one additional difference between FDA-approved drugs and dietary supplements. Methods for evaluating the exact composition of a drug and reporting this on the label and package insert is rigidly controlled by the FDA for all approved medicines, including generic drugs. It should be noted that generic drugs must meet the added burden of proving that they possess the same pharmacological properties as the name-brand drug for which they are intended to substitute. In contrast, while ingredients must be reported on the labels of food supplements, evaluating the purity and amounts of ingredients is left up to the manufacturer—without FDA supervision. For this reason, you do not have the same assurance as you would with an FDA-approved drug that the ingredients listed on the label of a dietary supplement are actually present or as pure as they should be.

The possible dangers of lack of FDA control were underscored by recent cases of lead poisoning from the use of herbal remedies imported from China, East India, Pakistan, and Latin America. Recently, the Centers for Disease Control reported the case of a woman who apparently developed elevated levels of lead in her blood from taking a Chinese herbal medication to control menstrual cramps. Lead, not listed as an ingredient in this remedy, is a potent neurotoxin—a poison that kills brain cells.

TESTING DRUGS TO IMPROVE MEMORY AND COGNITIVE FUNCTIONING

One strategy that has been used in determining the effectiveness of many of the drugs, including herbs and dietary supplements, that are discussed in this book has been to evaluate effectiveness in persons who are in the early stages of senility, either from Alzheimer's disease or other illnesses. The rationale for testing in such people is that since one of the primary symptoms of first-stage senility is forgetfulness, drugs that lessen these symptoms in such patients would surely improve the milder memory problems of otherwise healthy people. However, memory loss in senility is most likely due to the progressive death of neurons while forgetfulness in neurologically normal people probably results from other causes (a topic discussed in the next chapter). Therefore it is possible that drugs which are beneficial to persons suffering the symptoms of senility will not improve the memory of healthy people and vice versa.

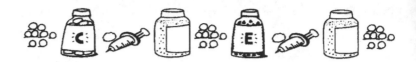

2

"Why Can't I Remember?"
The Effects of Biology, Genetics, and Environment on the Brain

While many people are fond of saying that the brain is similar to a computer, this analogy is somewhat misleading. Unlike a computer, which is made up of silicon chips and energized by electricity, the brain is a biological machine made up of neurons, living cells that are fed by substances in the blood and affected by what we eat, breathe, and feel. Because neurons are, in a sense, alive, the operations of the brain, including the ability to remember, are affected by scores of influences that have no effect on a computer. And with life comes both good and bad news. The bad news is that certain aspects of your lifestyle can interfere with your ability to perform well. The good news is that there may be practical steps you can take that will improve your mental abilities.

MEMORY AND MOOD: HOW EMOTIONS AFFECT BRAIN POWER

Depression is the emotion with the strongest effects on memory and other cognitive abilities. Unfortunately, its effect is negative. Functions impaired by depression include:

- Memory
- Attention and concentration
- Speed of thinking
- Posture and speed of movement
- Abstract thought and reasoning

There are many ways in which depression can have an impact on brain functioning. For example, depression frequently disrupts sleeping patterns. Researchers have discovered that the integrity of certain phases of sleep is crucial for memory to be stored adequately. Depression also causes a number of changes in the concentrations of various hormones. For example, the level of hormones secreted by the adrenal glands (the glucocorticoids) often increases with depression. Raised glucocorticoid levels interfere with memory storage and retrieval. Depression also causes large changes in the concentrations of neurotransmitters, the chemical messengers used by neurons to communicate with each other and process information. Changes of this type have a deleterious effect on the brain's ability to function efficiently.

Another strong influence on cognitive abilities is the reaction brought on by what is probably one of the most pervasive negative influences in our lives: stress. Research using laboratory animals has shown that severe stress can actually result in the death of brain cells. An area of the brain that is particularly sensitive to the effects of stress is called the hippocampus and is known to be involved in the formation of memory. Brain scans have shown that some people who have been exposed to severe and unremitting stress have decreased hippocampal volume. Even less severe stress has been shown in research studies to have a negative impact on cognitive abilities, although most probably the effect is not permanent.

Not surprisingly, in contrast to the negative effects of depression and stress, feelings of well-being seem to have beneficial effects on cognition. Positive mood appears to have both indirect and direct effects. Since, other factors being equal, positive mood results in fewer illnesses with consequent lower probability of medications that could compromise thinking abilities, this would indirectly improve cognition. In addition, research concerning the beneficial effects of certain drugs on learning ability have shown that while these drugs have no influences on memory per se, their beneficial cognitive influence stems from their ability to induce feelings of well-being. Based on this, it is plausible that positive mood directly facilitates learning and memory.

THE EFFECTS OF BODY CHEMISTRY ON YOUR MIND

Chemical messengers called hormones that are secreted into the blood by glands control the body's metabolism, its ability to consume energy. There are several hormones that have direct impact on cognitive processes, such as estrogen, androgens, thyroid, and glucocorticoid hormones. This is how each of these hormones influences brain functioning:

Estrogen and Androgens

Estrogen and androgens directly influence cognitive abilities in the following ways: Estrogen is produced in the ovaries in females and in the testes in men. Men normally have about one-fifth the level of estrogen as that found in a woman. In females, estrogens affect the growth and operation of the sexual organs, the fallopian tubes, and the development of secondary sexual characteristics (i.e., areas of fat deposit and hair growth). Estrogens in females also affect metabolism, bone growth, electrolyte balance, and neurotransmitter function in the brain. In males, estrogen's functions are unknown. Decreases in estrogen levels when women go through menopause are associated with problems in memory and abstract reasoning. Some postmenopausal cognitive deficits such as in verbal and visual memory, attention, and abstract reasoning may be improved or even reversed by estrogen replacement therapy.

Androgens (male sex hormones) including testosterone, dihydrotestosterone, and androstenedione (of Mark McGwire fame) are produced by the testes and, in both males and females, the adrenal glands. Androgens in males direct the development of the sexual organs and the secondary sexual characteristics, such as the deepening of the voice and hair distribution, as well as bone growth, muscular development, and metabolism. Apparently, one of the effects of androgens on cognitive functions is the enhancement of verbal fluency.

Thyroid Hormones

The thyroid hormone, which is produced by the thyroid gland, controls the body's metabolism. Low levels of thyroid hormones in developing children can result in cretinism, a condition associated with mental retardation. We know that thyroid hormone has a beneficial effect on the formation of memory. In addition, hypothyroidism (deficient production of thyroid hormone) causes depression which, in turn, negatively affects many aspects of cognition (see above).

Glucocorticoids

Glucocorticoids mainly affect carbohydrate, protein, and fat metabolism. Very high levels of these hormones impair our ability to retrieve information previously stored in long-term memory. Hydrocortisone, also known as cortisol, is the most common type of hormone secreted by the adrenal glands in response to stress, trauma of any kind, extreme cold or heat, infection, or virtually any disease. In addition, cortisol is an extremely effective anti-inflammatory agent but, at the same time, it impairs the functioning of the immune system.

THE WORLD WE LIVE IN: ELECTROMAGNETIC WAVES, MSG, AND ALUMINUM POTS

There are a variety of agents in the environment that have been suggested to have a negative impact on people's ability to think. Electromagnetic waves (electrical fields); monosodium glutamate (MSG), which can cause what is known—even in medical journals—as the Chinese restaurant syndrome; aluminum (absorbed through drinking water, pots, cans, and deodorant); and lead (ingested as lead paint dust and from old pipes with lead solder joints) are the usual suspects.

Electromagnetic Waves

For some time there has been a suspicion that the electrical fields surrounding high voltage lines have deleterious effects on people living nearby. Electromagnetic waves from cell phones, electric blankets, and other household appliances have also been held suspect. The most common effect is thought to be an increase in leukemia and other cancers, particularly in children. The relationship to leukemia has been intensively studied over the past decade and has resulted in passionate debate but no resolution. Although most scientific opinion suggests that there is no effect, a recent review of these studies concluded: "Even if there is no currently understood biological plausibility for such an association, its possible causal nature cannot be dismissed. The impact on public health of such a possible causal association is difficult to assess precisely but could be significant."

If it's even in the realm of possibility that electromagnetic waves affect the body sufficiently to trigger cancers, is it also possible that they can affect the brain? There have been a number of studies of the effects of electrical fields on animals' ability to learn, and in all cases, fields disrupted learning and memory. However, before starting to worry, one should be aware of several important points. First, the strength of the fields used in many of the experimental studies was far in excess of those experienced by most people out in the real world. Second, it is not known if weaker fields, similar to those experienced by people living near high voltage lines, would affect learning in animals since no studies have yet been published using lower intensity fields. Third, although there have been a few studies of the effects of living near high tension lines on cognitive functions of people, there's no agreement on whether there are significant influences. One could draw some comfort from the knowledge that the high-intensity pulsed electrical fields associated with Magnetic Resonance Imaging (MRI), though far stronger than fields from high voltage cables, appear to have no detrimental effects. On the other hand, fields caused by MRIs differ from the steady state electromagnetic waves surrounding high-tension lines.

MSG—Monosodium Glutamate

Similar to the effects of electromagnetic waves, there is also controversy among scientists as to the effects, if any, of MSG. Although MSG does not affect everybody, people who believe that they are sensitive to this food additive describe similar symptoms: headaches, muscle tightness, general weakness, skin flushing, and mental fog. Until recently, the weight of scientific opinion was that "Chinese restaurant syndrome is an anecdote applied to a variety of postprandial illnesses; rigorous and realistic scientific evidence linking the syndrome to MSG could not be found." Following on the heels of this pronouncement that appeared to strike the death knell of the Chinese restaurant syndrome came a study providing the aforementioned "rigorous and realistic scientific evidence." In a double-blind placebo-controlled study, "MSG reproduced symptoms in alleged sensitive persons." Based on this finding, it was concluded that "the symptoms, originally called the Chinese restaurant syndrome, are better referred to as the MSG symptom complex."

Studies of MSG in laboratory animals, using the usual super-colossal doses common to most experiments of this kind, showed the expected disruption of learning and memory. Convincing studies in humans are yet to be conducted. However, if the existence of a monosodium glutamate symptom complex can be verified, people who are sensitive to this food additive can, after consuming a meal rich in MSG, expect at least a temporary effect on thinking ability.

Aluminum

In the 1960s, Dr. Henry Wisniewski and his colleagues discovered that when aluminum was injected into the brains of rabbits, certain changes developed that resembled some of the pathology (neurofibrillary tangles) seen in Alzheimer's disease. Shortly thereafter, another scientist, Dr. Donald Crapper-McLachlan, performed autopsies on Alzheimer's patients and reported that he found aluminum in their brains. With this was born the "aluminum hypothesis" of Alzheimer's disease, which asserted that exposure to aluminum caused Alzheimer's. Unfortunately, like most simple solutions to complex problems, this easy explanation for Alzheimer's proved to be incorrect. Following his discovery that aluminum produced tangles in rabbit brains, Dr. Wisniewski found that these tangles were only superficially similar to those seen in Alzheimer's and, even more disappointing, did not occur in other animals, including humans. In addition, recent work suggests that whatever aluminum accumulates in the brains of Alzheimer's patients is most likely caused by the disease rather than the reverse.

BLAME IT ON YOUR PARENTS: THE ROLE OF GENETICS

Some people seem to stay young forever (without benefit of plastic surgery) while others appear to age before our eyes. The rate at which different people change as they grow older is most likely the product of a complex interaction between the influences of a multitude of genes and a myriad of environmental factors. Genetics clearly play an important role in directly determining an individual's cognitive abilities as well as controlling other factors that ultimately affect that person's cognitive abilities (e.g., the brain's capacity to resist injury). However, there are a variety of other factors that fall under the general rubric of environmental influences that have equally strong effects on the development of intellectual abilities. The overlapping and complimentary roles of genetics and environment, often called "nature/nurture," is graphically illustrated by studies of the IQs of identical twins. Although initially the IQs of the siblings are highly correlated, as they age their IQs become increasingly dissimilar. Since identical twins have identical genetic makeup, the progressive changes with aging reflect the accumulating influences of environment.

One gene that has attracted a lot of attention in recent research is involved in the brain's ability to withstand the effects of aging and other potentially damaging influences. This gene, called apolipoprotein E (APO-E), comes in at least three forms, or alleles: APO-E2, APO-E3, and APO-

E4. People who carry two copies of APO-E4 have a significantly increased risk of developing Alzheimer's disease. In addition, even in the absence of Alzheimer's disease, these people tend to develop memory problems as they grow older. Furthermore, people with this genetic makeup also tend to show less recovery from traumatic brain injury.

In addition to APO-E4, other genes have been identified that can affect whether or not a person will develop Alzheimer's disease. In particular, the presence of the presenilin gene virtually guarantees the early development of Alzheimer's disease. Fortunately, very few in the general population are carrying this booby-trapped DNA in their genetic makeup. There are, however, other genes in addition to the presenilin gene that affect the brain's response to aging. For example, people with Down's syndrome almost always develop Alzheimer's disease in middle age. Some researchers think that a form of the genetic defect that produces Down's syndrome, an abnormality on the twenty-first chromosome, may also lead to the development of senile dementia in some people without Down's syndrome.

Although genetics are important in determining brain power and the effects of aging, one should not despair; biology is not destiny. The environment, specifically the activities in which an individual chooses to participate, can have a powerful effect on cognition and resistance to the potentially deleterious effects of getting older. Epidemiological studies have made three important facts abundantly clear. First, the more education a person has, the less the cognitive decline with increasing age. Second, although the brain appears to get smaller with advancing age, individuals with more education show smaller decreases in brain size as they get older. Third, in persons destined to develop Alzheimer's disease, there are indications that previous education or simply engaging in activities that cause you to think will delay the onset of the illness by years.

Unfortunately, these studies suffer from the chicken-or-the-egg dilemma in that it is unclear whether there are beneficial effects of education or, conversely, if those who are resistant to aging effects have the type of brain that make these people more likely to go to school and to engage in cognitively challenging careers. Research using laboratory animals strongly supports the idea that it is education or engaging in activities that cause you to think that has beneficial effects on the survival of your brain power. When two groups of rats that were genetically similar were raised in dramatically different environments, examination of their brains after they became adults revealed important differences. The brains of rats that were raised in "enriched" environments, areas with toys, tunnels, and activity wheels, were larger and heavier than the brains of siblings raised in impoverished environments. Microscopic examination of the brain cells of the rats from the enriched environment revealed highly complex branching not seen in their deprived brethren. In addition, other studies have shown that brain cells from rats that were raised in enriched environments are much less likely to die when exposed to certain toxic substances.

BETTER LIVING THROUGH CHEMISTRY? THE NEGATIVE INFLUENCES OF SOME PRESCRIPTION AND RECREATIONAL DRUGS

As you will learn in the next chapter, the normal activity of brain cells (neurons) is dependent on complex chemical reactions that allow these living computing devices to process information accurately and efficiently. Because the actions of neurons are chemically dependent, altering that chemistry can either enhance or impair their ability to process information. Unfortunately, it seems that it is far easier to change brain chemistry in such a way as to diminish thinking power than it is to improve it.

Many drugs, both prescription medications and over-the-counter remedies, have negative influences on cognitive abilities. Among the most commonly prescribed drugs are anxiolytics, minor tranquilizers such as Valium, used to dull the ever-present effects of stress. People who take such tranquilizers commonly score lower on tests of memory than their less tranquil counterparts. As already described, depression has a strong negative impact on a variety of cognitive processes. However, the drugs often necessary to treat depression can have their own set of adverse effects on thinking ability, including problems with memory and attention. For those people who really need either tranquilizers or antidepressants, it is likely that the deleterious effects of anxiety or depression on their cognitive abilities far outweigh the adverse effects of the medications. However, it must be recognized that these drugs have negative effects as well; the risk/benefit ratio discussed in Chapter 1 rears its head.

While it is understandable that tranquilizers and antidepressants, drugs designed to act on the brain, can interfere with thinking ability, it is surprising that many other drugs that are not intended to affect the brain also can alter cognition. Most recently a great deal of attention has been directed toward the effects of aspirin and nonsteroidal anti-inflammatory drugs (NSAIDs) (such as ibuprofen). Drugs of this type are widely used to combat headache and arthritis pain as well as pain and discomfort from fever, overexertion, and any of the myriad other noxious influences in day-to-day living. The story concerning aspirin and NSAIDs is complex and, since research is currently under way, still unfolding. Early research indicated that people who took these drugs every day had a lower incidence of Alzheimer's disease. Based on this, it was hypothesized that the anti-inflammatory effects of these agents counteracted the brain swelling that accompanies the disease process in Alzheimer's and that is in part responsible for the death of brain cells. By reducing inflammation in the brain, aspirin and NSAIDs were thought to slow down the rate at which neurons died and thereby delay the appearance of Alzheimer's symptoms. In addition to anti-inflammatory properties, these drugs have also been shown to act as antioxidants. Since oxidative stress is also thought to be one of the routes by which brain cells are killed in Alzheimer's disease, the antioxidant effects of aspirin and NSAIDs were thought to be another way that these drugs protected the brain from the ravages of Alzheimer's disease. Unfortunately, aspirin and NSAID use appears to conform to what seems to be a universal rule in biology if not life in general: Too much of a good thing is not a good thing. While chronic use of low doses of these drugs seems to have beneficial effects, particularly in older people, repeated use of higher doses is associated with a decline in cognitive abilities. Again, however, we have a chicken-or-the-egg type of problem in interpreting these results. It is possible that high doses of these drugs do in fact negatively impact the brain or, conversely, that people who take higher doses require more medication because they are in poor health and it is the illness that impairs their cognitive abilities rather than the medication.

The list of drugs that can have a negative influence on cognition is long and, as with most drugs, there are differences in the susceptibility of particular individuals to specific medication effects. A recent article listed fifty-five commonly used drugs, both prescription and over-the-counter, that can cause disorientation. Included were commonly used treatments for mood disorders, heart disease, hypertension, and allergy problems. A list of equivalent length was included for drugs that could cause depression, which can adversely affect thinking ability (see above).

In addition to the effects of prescription and over-the-counter drugs, other chemicals that some of us ingest for entertainment purposes (i.e., recreational drugs such as alcohol, cocaine, marijuana) affect the brain and in so doing alter cognitive abilities. The most commonly used drug, alcohol, also appears to be potentially the most damaging to the brain. Chronic alcoholism, if it continues long enough, can result in widespread damage to the brain. This damage can include reduction in overall size, presumably through loss of neurons, and more specific damage in the frontal lobes (involved in higher level executive functions), hippocampus (important for memory formation), and cerebellum (involved in control of movements). Not surprisingly, alcoholism is associated with a variety of cognitive problems including impaired learning ability, memory, and problem-solving ability. If an alcoholic abstains and the previous period of drinking had not gone on too long, these cognitive problems slowly resolve over a period of up to five years. Unfortunately, if you drink alcoholic beverages and are not an alcoholic, you are not necessarily in the clear; social drinkers can also show lasting aftereffects of ingesting alcohol. According to current research, "persons drinking five or six U.S. standard drinks per day over extended time periods manifest some cognitive inefficiencies; at seven to nine drinks per day, mild cognitive deficits are present; and at 10 or more drinks per day, moderate cognitive deficits equivalent to those found in diagnosed alcoholics are present."*

Other recreational drugs also can have effects on cognition. Cocaine impairs cognitive functioning even in those who cannot be classified as addicts. The brains of "casual" users show areas of abnormally decreased blood flow or oxygen consumption even six months after their last drug use. These same people had impaired attention, learning, and memory abilities. Similar findings have also been reported for people who use either amphetamine type drugs or less traditional drugs such as Ecstasy. In contrast, despite extensive research there is no solid evidence of any lasting aftereffects of marijuana use, even in those who could be considered to be heavy users. The jury is still out, however, concerning the possibility that marijuana use has more subtle residual effects on cognition.

THE AGING BRAIN

In the Western world few people view the prospect of growing older with optimism or enthusiasm. It is still widely believed that we are all faced with a progressive and inevitable waning of our mental powers in association with an accelerating loss of brain cells as we gradually slide into doddering senescence. Fortunately, current research indicates that

---

*O. A. Parsons and S. J. Nixon, "Cognitive Functioning in Sober Social Drinkers: A Review of the Research since 1986. *Journal of the Study of Alcohol* 59(2): 180–90, 1998.

aging is not necessarily associated with such a depressing outcome.

If the subjects used for the studies of cognition and the brain during aging are confined to healthy individuals, the long-term picture is much more positive. There are indeed age-related declines in memory power but of a lesser degree and more restricted than was formerly believed. Acquisition and immediate retrieval of new information was negatively impacted by aging, but long-term retention was not affected. In addition, other aspects of cognitive functioning, including language ability, visuospatial perceptual functions, and abstract reasoning, were not adversely affected by aging.

The problem for most of us, unfortunately, is that the odds of maintaining excellent heath into old age, if not a long shot, are still not in our favor. Stress plus age-related declines in the functioning of many of our bodily systems leave us increasingly open to a variety of ailments that could ultimately affect cognitive powers. For example, hypertension frequently develops in middle age and is often treated with beta blockers. Beta blockers can induce depression, which, in turn, can adversely affect cognitive powers. Other drugs used to treat noncognitive disorders can also have a direct negative influence on our thinking ability. For example, a recent paper lists fifty-five commonly used medications, including an antibiotic, antihistamines, anti-inflammatory agents, and some cardiovascular drugs, that can produce disorientation. The potential problem is magnified since many people have to take several drugs ("polypharmacy") that may interact in undocumented and unpredictable ways. In addition to the deleterious effects of drugs used to treat ailments associated with aging, certain medical conditions in and of themselves can have negative effects. For example, atrial fibrillation, a disorder affecting the beating of one of the heart's four chambers, does not usually result in problems such as a heart attack or heart failure. However, due to the inefficient pumping action of the heart during episodes of arrthymia, the brain does not get enough oxygen and, if untreated, this condition weakens our memory and other cognitive abilities. There are a host of other diseases and medicines used in their treatment that are all-too-common companions of our old age and that can, either independently or in concert, decrease our cognitive abilities.

In addition to the medical problems of aging, the changes in lifestyle that are often associated with retirement can also cause problems. Engaging in activities that make us use our brains, such as reading books or learning a new skill or sport, seems to protect neurons from the multitude of influences that can adversely affect their functioning. Retirement, and the release from the responsibilities associated with employment, can free us sufficiently to engage in such activities. Unfortunately, it also allows us to sit in front of a television and veg out, so that cognitive powers will in all likelihood wane.

If you wish to maintain your cognitive abilities, your course is clear. Don't age or get sick, avoid drugs (prescription, over-the-counter, and recreational), read really great books, avoid stress, be happy, and, equally important, pick parents with good genetic makeup. Those unable to follow this simple recipe will, to some extent, experience the effects of aging, and the remaining chapters of this book are for them.

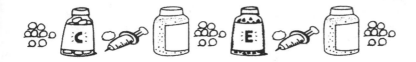

Chemistry and the Brain:
Why Drugs Can Help You Think Better

The incredible power of the human brain was graphically demonstrated in the chess matches between the supercomputer Big Blue and the world chess champion, Garry Kasparov. Big Blue, which is actually made up of thirty-two computers working in unison, can consider two hundred million chess positions each second. However, despite this phenomenal power to calculate, the computer was decisively beaten by the human—in their first short match. As a result, Big Blue was radically overhauled and made even more powerful before meeting Kasparov for a second match. In their second contest, Kasparov was finally beaten, but only by the barest of margins. What enables an approximately two-pound mass of living tissue to accomplish such tasks, to compose music, write books, love, hate, or mediate any of the innumerable acts that are routinely performed by humans? The basis of the brain's enormous capacities resides in the unique ability of its cells to communicate with each other via electrochemical reactions. This chapter will explain the basic biological mechanisms that lie at the heart of neuronal communication and why there is a plausible rationale for the use of drugs to enhance cognitive abilities.

Neurons

Like all cells, neurons have a cell body with a nucleus containing DNA that regulates all of the neuron's activities, energy generating machinery, and a variety of organelles that synthesize all of the substances needed to maintain normal functioning. However, neurons also have a variety of specializations that allow them to act as the biological equivalent of miniature computers.

FIGURE 1.

A schematic drawing of two neurons illustrating their basic components. Dendrite: tapering projections from the cell body (also called soma); axon: a thinner projection from the cell body that barely tapers; axon terminal: an enlargement at the end; synapse: the area of close apposition between two neurons (1 and 2) wherein an axon terminal is closely adjacent to a dendrite or cell body of another neuron.

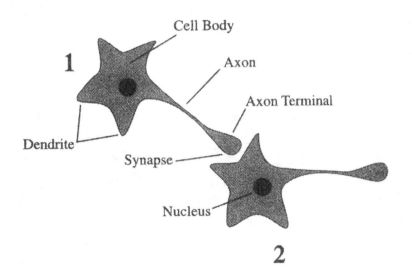

COMMUNICATION BETWEEN NEURONS

Neurons are designed to conduct electrical impulses. When a neuron is activated (Figure 2), an electrical impulse rapidly travels from the area of the dendrites and cell body, to the axon and then along the axon to its terminal. When the electrical discharge reaches the axon terminal, the impulse affects the adjacent neuron on the other side of the synapse. In the majority of cases, the electrical impulse does not jump across the gap in the synapse as is often depicted in cartoons and science fiction movies. Most communication between neurons depends on chemical messengers called neurotransmitters.

FIGURE 2.

This figure shows the passage of electric activity from one neuron (at left) to another (at right). The same two neurons are shown in A–D as time elapses. A. A dendrite of the neuron at the left is activated (white area) by another brain cell that is not shown in the figure. B. The activation travels into the cell body, a process taking about one millisecond (one one thousandth of a second). C. The electrical impulse travels down the axon. D. The electrical activity from the neuron at the left causes activation of the neuron at the right.

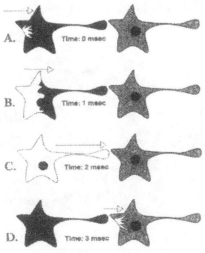

Neurotransmitters

Neurotransmitters are chemicals stored in spherical packets, called synaptic vesicles, that are, in turn, located in axon terminals (Figure 3). When a neuron is activated and the electrical impulse travels down into the terminal, the synaptic vesicles open and dump their chemical contents through pores into the synapse. The neurotransmitters float across the gap between the neurons and contact the adjacent dendrite or cell body, causing an electrical response. The area contacted by the neurotransmitters is different from other parts of the neuron and is designed to respond electrically to that specific neurotransmitter. This target of the neurotransmitter is called the receptor.

FIGURE 3.

This figure is a simplified schematic of a synapse. The synapse, the area of close apposition between the axon terminal of neuron 1 and the soma of neuron 2 (within the circle), is magnified in the cross-sectional view. Spherical synaptic vesicles store molecules of chemical neurotransmitters. When the neuron is activated and electrical activity enters the axon terminal, the vesicles open and expel their chemical contents out from the terminal into the space (called the synaptic cleft) between neurons 1 and 2. When the transmitter molecules diffuse across the cleft and contact neuron 2 at the receptor, these chemicals triger an electrical response in that brain cell.

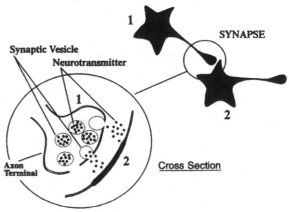

There are at least one hundred different chemicals that act as neurotransmitters. Different neurotransmitters are often located in different parts of the brain and have unique kinds of effects on the neurons that they contact. In general, a neurotransmitter can either activate a neuron or shut it down. Neurotransmitters that activate are termed excitatory and those that suppress are called inhibitory.

Neurons as Mini-Computers

The biological properties of neurons allow them to integrate and store enormous volumes of information. Let's look at how a neuron handles information, using basic computer terms with which we are all familiar.

NEURON ACTIVITY = INFORMATION

Everything that you know about your environment has been translated by your brain into the language of neurons-electrochemical activity. Light from the objects you see affects photosensitive chemicals in specialized visual receptor cells in the retina that subsequently trigger electrical impulses in the nerve that carries that information into your brain. Similarly, when you touch something, the pressure on your skin squeezes somatosensory receptor cells that activate sensory nerves, initiating impulses that travel to your brain. If you decide to pick up what you have touched, first that decision has to be made in executive portions of your brain by neurons that arrive at and signal their conclusion by firing impulses to motor areas that will activate your spinal cord again via nerve impulses. The motor areas in your spinal cord fire impulses down their axons targeting the appropriate muscles that will contract in response to the nerve activity and grasp the object to be picked up.

FIGURE 4

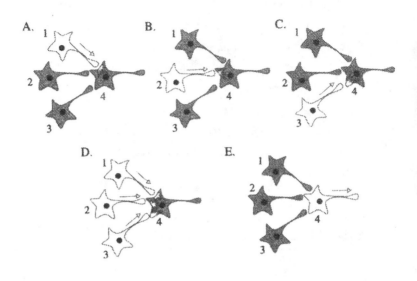

INTEGRATION OF INFORMATION

The activity of one neuron will rarely, if ever, cause the activation of a second neuron. This is illustrated in Figure 4, where a four-neuron circuit is shown. In A, neuron 1 fires but causes only a sub-threshold activation of neuron 4, which is insufficient to trigger an impulse down its axon. In B, neuron 2 fires but also causes only a sub-threshold activation of neuron 4, while in C, neuron 3 is similarly ineffective in fully activating neuron 4. In D, however, neurons 1, 2, and 3 fire together and their synchronous activity is summed in neuron 4 to a level that is sufficient to cause full activation, as illustrated in E.

Neurons function as integrators because they require synchronous activation from many other neurons to be activated. In reality, there are influences from excitatory neurotransmitters that push a neuron toward full activation, and also influences from inhibitory neurotransmitters that tend to counteract the excitatory neurotransmitters. A neuron's activity at any instant in time is determined by the sum of the inhibitory and excitatory influences. The number of influences that affect a neuron's activity is enormous. There are from 10,000 to 100,000 synapses on each neuron and there are about 200 billion neurons in the adult human brain.

FIGURE 5.

Brain areas involved in memory. A. The four lobes of the brain. B. Parts of the cortex that become activated during a memory task. C. View of the brain in which the frontal cortex and the temporal cortex have been removed to reveal two additional structures involved in memory: the hippocampus and striatum.

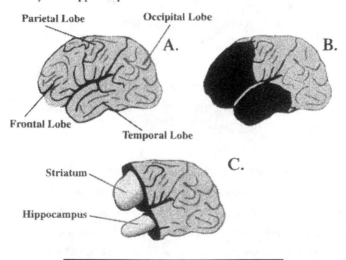

INFORMATION STORAGE

Many neurons are designed in such a way that they will learn from past experience and remember. For example, if an event is often associated with the firing of a given neuron, it gradually becomes easier and easier for that event to activate the neuron—this is how repetitive behaviors, or habits, are formed. The processes that enable a neuron to "profit from experience" are the subject of intensive scientific research and are only now just beginning to be understood. Among the changes that occur when a neuron "learns" is the production of more neurotransmitter, physical alteration of the synapse that allows it to be more easily affected by neurotransmitters, the growth of new synapses, changes in messenger RNA, generation of new proteins, and a laundry list of other cellular modifications that enhance the ability of a brain cell to respond to important inputs.

Although the majority of neurons have the ability to change their activity based on past experience, brain cells that learn most easily are often located in parts of the brain that are specialized to form and store a person's memories. In the past it was thought that there were memory areas in the brain much in the same sense that computers have storage devices such as hard drives and floppy discs. Indeed, damage in certain parts of the brain, most notably a structure called the hippocampus (see Figure 5C), produced severe and lasting disturbances of certain aspects of the patient's ability to remember or learn. More recently, however, it has been discovered that there are no memory areas per se; instead, there are memory systems made up of a number of interconnected parts of the brain that must function in synchrony in order for information to be stored and retrieved when necessary. For example, in experiments in which the activation of a patient's brain could be observed through the use of a technique called functional magnetic resonance imaging (functional MRI), a simple act of memorization involved the frontal lobes, cerebellum, hippocampus, striatum, and other structures (Figure 5).

Like the brain systems that store information, memory itself is a complex, multilayered process. An idea of the complicated nature of memory is illustrated in numerous case histories of patients who have suffered some form of brain injury. One of the best documented is that of a patient referred to by the initials H.M. This man suffered from epileptic attacks that, at the time (1954), were not responsive to any available drug treatment. Since the seizures were totally disabling, it was decided to remove the part of the brain wherein the epilepsy appeared to originate, the temporal lobes. Following the surgery H.M. evidenced no changes in personality or reasoning ability. Indeed, his IQ actually increased, probably due to the decrease in the frequency of epileptic seizures. However, removal of H.M.'s temporal lobes was not without effect; immediately following the surgery and persisting to the present day, he suffers from an incapacitating and singular type of memory problem. Although his memory of events preceding the surgery is intact, H.M. is unable to remember for very long anything of his life following surgery. "The central feature of his amnesia continues to be a failure in long-term retention for most ongoing events. This forgetfulness applies to the surroundings of the house where he has lived for the past six years, and to those neighbors who have been visiting the house regularly during this period. He has not yet learned their names and does not recognize them if he meets them in the street."* He can remember their names for a few minutes after being introduced but soon forgets and has to be reintroduced again. The process is repeated with each suc-

---

*B. Milner, "Memory and the Medial Temporal Regions of the Brain." In *The Biology of Memory*, New York: Academic Press, 1970, pp. 29–50.

cessive encounter, not only with people, but also all events of life. Thus, while H.M.'s recollection of the past (i.e., long-term memory) and his ability to remember things such as a person's name for a few minutes is intact, his ability to store new information in long-term memory was precluded by the loss of his temporal lobes.

Clearly, memory cannot be considered to be a unitary process. Research and examination of patients with brain injury has identified a number of processes that together function as memory (illustrated in Figure 6). Procedural memory refers to those highly practiced and ingrained behaviors, such as buttoning your shirt, that one does automatically with little or no conscious thought. Such memories are extremely durable and are adversely affected by only the most catastrophic brain injury. Declarative memory encompasses virtually all other types of memory and is subdivided into semantic and episodic categories. Semantic memory is the storage of basic facts while episodic is the storage of events. For example, the knowledge that 1:00 A.M is one o'clock in the morning is semantic memory while recollection of what you did at 1:00 A.M. is episodic memory. Storage of both semantic and also episodic memory is a two-stage process in which information passes through temporary storage (short-term memory) into a more permanent storage (long-term memory). Short-term memory is extremely fragile and susceptible to disruption by any of a variety of influences, such as drugs, alcohol, or head injury, while long-term memory, like procedural memory, is invulnerable to all but the most serious forms of brain injury or disease.

Another form of memory is distinguished by the fact that, by design, it is of short duration. This type of brain process, called working memory, keeps information available only for a finite time, during which it can be used to guide behavior. An example of working memory is the ability to remember a phone number told to you by the directory assistance operator long enough to dial it.

Finally, there is another division of memory processes that must be considered. Verbal information, spoken language, and information gained by reading, is processed by the left half or hemisphere of the brain, while information that is seen, but not converted into words, is processed by the right hemisphere.

FIGURE 6.

Processes that function as memory.

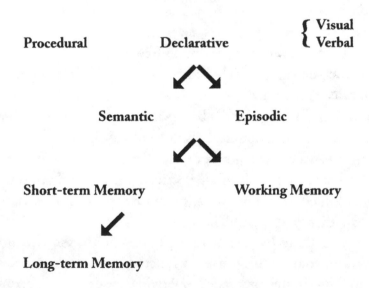

It should be recognized that the ability of your memory systems to function efficiently depends on many factors, some of which—mood, alcohol use, hormone levels—were discussed in the preceding chapter. Another important influence on memory is your ability to pay attention, to focus on the relevant while warding off distraction caused by the irrelevant. Frequently, people who have suffered a head injury that disrupts the brain's attention systems experience their symptoms as memory problems. The success of treatments of attentional problems, for example by use of Ritalin in some children with attention deficit disorder, is reflected in improvements in learning ability.

HOW DRUGS HAVE THEIR EFFECTS: WHY DRUGS MAY HELP YOU THINK BETTER

Every aspect of a neuron's functioning depends on chemicals. Communication between neurons is accomplished by the brain's chemical messengers, neurotransmitters. The electrical activity of neurons, the maximum frequency of a neuron's firing, and the speed at which impulses travel down the axon, are all determined by a host of chemical reactions. Information storage by the brain's memory neurons is accomplished by a variety of changes in neuronal chemistry, including increases in the amount of neurotransmitter squirted into the synapse as a result of an electrical impulse and prolongation of the duration of excitation caused by a transmitter.

In theory, it should be possible to improve the brain's ability to think by taking drugs that enhance the chemical reactions that a neuron uses to function or to store information. This is the rationale underlying treatment of certain brain disorders such as Parkinson's disease. In Parkinson's disease, neurons that use a neurotransmitter called dopamine, in an area of the brain that controls movement, die. As a result, persons with this disease develop symptoms such as tremors, difficulty beginning a movement, and balance problems. To treat Parkinson's, a substance called L-DOPA is administered, the brain converts L-DOPA to dopamine, and some of the patient's symptoms lessen. Some scientists think that as a person ages, there is a progressive decrease in the concentration of certain neurotransmitters that are used by memory neurons. If this is true, it is reasonable to assume that administering drugs that restore the levels of these transmitters would stave off age-related memory loss. Similarly, it should be possible to counteract the deleterious effects of illness, stress, prescription drugs, and a host of other influences on thinking ability by administering drugs that increase the activity of chemicals used by neurons to function efficiently.

Unfortunately, there may be a fly in the ointment. The nature of the problem is illustrated by the effects of trying to restore dopamine levels in patients with Parkinson's disease. As already mentioned, the patient's symptoms lessen when dopamine levels are brought back to near-normal levels by the administration of L-DOPA. So what is the problem? Despite the fact that dopamine levels are increased, the *patient* remains far from normal. The symptoms of Parkinson's disease include movement problems, already mentioned, and cognitive impairments. Although motor symptoms are less severe after the restoration of dopamine, cognitive symptoms may not be affected or may actually worsen. In addition, after several years of treatment, administration of L-DOPA begins to elicit abnormal movements that are as disabling as the symptoms of Parkinson's disease.

There are two important questions that can be asked in connection with the effects of L-DOPA.

1. First, why is it that L-DOPA not only does not cure Parkinson's disease but also causes problems of its own?

2. Two, what is the relevance to the use of drugs to improve cognition?

The reason L-DOPA is given to Parkinson's disease patients is to partially restore dopamine levels. However, in normal persons, dopamine is stored in brain cells in a particular area, this neurotransmitter is released in a tightly controlled fashion by the activity of those neurons, and the concentrations of available dopamine are precisely regulated by biochemical mechanisms in the brain. When dopamine levels are controlled by the external administration of L-DOPA, none of these processes is in effect. The dopamine produced by conversion of L-DOPA cannot be targeted for only those brain areas where it has been depleted by disease, its release is not regulated by neuronal activity, and its concentration in any area of the brain is not regulated by the brain's biochemical mechanisms. For these reasons it is not surprising that L-DOPA does not make patients with Parkinson's disease completely normal.

The relevance of all this to you, the consumer, is that the rationale underlying the use of L-DOPA in Parkinson's (i.e., restoration of declining dopamine levels) is identical to the rationale for the use of other drugs to improve cognition. When taking a drug that affects concentrations of neurotransmitters in the brain, the purported mode of action of many of the food supplements advertised as cognition-enhancers, one must consider the possibility of unexpected and sometimes adverse effects.

For this reason it is imperative to know as much as possible about a drug and its effects before putting it in your body. With a prescription medication, this is an easy task since there is a system for compiling relevant information on drug actions and side effects. However, despite the lack of FDA scrutiny of food supplements and herbs, there is considerable information in the medical and scientific journals concerning the actions of many of these drugs. The purpose of the following chapters is to summarize this information. In all cases it is strongly suggested that your decision to take a food supplement be discussed with a qualified health professional.

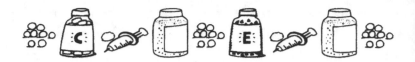

4

Smart Drugs and Nootropics

Although the terms *smart drug* and *nootropic* are often used interchangeably, they have slightly different meanings. A smart drug is any chemical substance that improves thinking abilities such as memory, attention, and abstract thought, but may also have other effects on other parts of the body as well. Often smart drugs were designed with other uses in mind but were found to have effects on cognitive abilities. On the other hand, a nootropic is a smart drug that was specifically designed to influence cognition and whose actions in the body are confined to effects on thinking. Thus, if a particular vitamin improves memory, it is a smart drug, but because it has a variety of other effects on the body, it is not a nootropic.

In this chapter, as in each of the following chapters in which specific drugs are discussed, we will review the claims made in support of a particular substance's beneficial effects, the theories put forth to explain its actions, the scientific evidence that the drug is effective, and the nature of side effects and other possible dangers, if any. In deciding whether to take a drug, the last two types of information are by far the most relevant.

ADRAFINIL
Nonprescription drug; available through Internet suppliers

What is it?

Adrafinil is a nonprescription drug that is sold in Europe under the brand name of Olmifon; it is not approved for use in the United States. It is used for the treatment of narcolepsy, a condition where the person experiences excessive daytime sleepiness and the propensity to fall asleep suddenly. Although the actions of this drug are not well understood, it is thought to belong to a class of drugs known as alpha-adrenergic agonists. Such drugs act by mimicking some of the effects of epinephrine, a hormone secreted by the adrenal gland in response to a variety of conditions including exercise and stress, and norepinephrine, a neurotransmitter that is released by neurons both in and outside the brain to affect bodily functions under the same circumstances as those that trigger adrenal release of epinephrine. The effects of epinephrine are diverse and include increases in heart rate, blood pressure, breathing rate, and metabolism. There are at least nine different types of receptors (receptors are explained in Figure 3, Chapter 3) for epinephrine and norepinephrine, called alpha 1A, alpha 1B, alpha 1D, alpha 2B, alpha 2C, beta 1, beta 2, and beta 3. Adrafinil is thought to work by activating only the alpha 1 types of receptor and thereby causes many unwanted reactions.

Its reputation

Adrafinil is promoted as a stimulant that energizes and increases attention without the agitation, anxiety, and sleeplessness associated with other stimulants such as caffeine, amphetamine, and cocaine. In addition to improving energy levels and concentration, this drug is also advanced as an aid to mental clarity and memory. It is suggested that the more benign profile of adrafinil, as compared to other stimulants, is due to its selective effects on the brain's alpha-adrenergic receptors. Other stimulants can affect both alpha and beta receptors as well as dopamine receptors.

The drug's effect on the brain

The effects of adrafinil in the brain are, for the most part, unknown. There is no direct evidence that this drug is an alpha 1 agonist; experiments in which adrafinil is observed binding to these or any other types of receptors have not been published. Its selective effect on alpha 1 receptors is inferred from indirect evidence that is not persuasive. In addition, it has been shown that, if adrafinil does not directly activate dopamine receptors, it certainly does affect dopamine indirectly.

Adrafinil clearly does act as a stimulant based on the results of studies in mice, rats, and monkeys. Whether or not this drug does not produce sleeplessness is questionable; adrafinil increased the activity of monkeys during the night to levels that were identical to those observed during the day. In addition, the activating effects of a single dose of adrafinil lasted thirty-six hours.

How has it been tested? What are the risks, if any?

A search through MEDLINE, the National Library of Medicine's bibliographic database, a listing of over 9.2 million articles from more than 3,800 international biomedical journals since 1966, did not turn up a single paper reporting the effects of adrafinil in people. Indeed, there were also no papers that described influences of this drug on attention, memory, or other cognitive abilities in laboratory animals.

The source of the reports of this drug's beneficial effects on cognition, its absence of side effects, and its overall safety, appear to be solely based on unverified anecdotes and on testimonials circulated by commercial suppliers.

In view of the lack of published testing in people, the risks of using adrafinil are largely unknown. The risks associated with other adrenergic agonists may be relevant to adrafinil and should be heeded in the absence of solid evidence indicating otherwise. The major side effect is elevation of blood pressure, an adverse event with potentially serious results in persons with hypertension and other cardiovascular illnesses. Other side effects are stomach pain, skin irritations, and elevated liver enzymes.

In addition to these effects of alpha adrenergic agonists, risks of stimulants in general should be considered. Many stimulants are exceedingly addictive; no data exists concerning this potential risk of adrafinil. This is particularly important since many addictive drugs activate dopamine receptors, an action that adrafinil appears to accomplish indirectly.

Typical dosages
Adrafinil is manufactured in 300 mg tablets. Typically, 600 to 1,200 mg is administered daily in divided doses.

Contraindications
Based on its known actions, this drug should not be taken by anyone with hypertension, cardiovascular disease, or insomnia. In addition, adrafinil has been shown to interact with yohimbine to increase effects, an adverse event that can result in toxicity. Accordingly, adrafinil should not be used by people taking supplements that contain yohimbine or the prescription drug Yokon.

The plain facts

Adrafinil lacks sufficient scientific documentation of its beneficial effects, side effects, or the nature of its actions. Due to this lack of information, the risks of using adrafinil clearly outweigh the known benefits.

Benefits: ½
Risks: 4

ALPHA-GPC
Dietary supplement; available over the counter

What is it?

Alpha-GPC, the abbreviation for alpha-glycerylphosphorylcholine, is thought to be used by the brain to increase the levels of choline that are, in turn, converted to the neurotransmitter acetylcholine.

Its reputation

Based upon its presumed action in increasing brain acetylcholine levels, alpha-GPC is advertised as a general memory enhancer.

The drug's effect on the brain

Although choline levels in the blood dramatically increase within an hour of ingesting alpha-GPC, do acetylcholine levels increase in the brain? Experiments involving rats indicate that as advertised, alpha-GPC does appear to increase acetylcholine levels in the cortex and hippocampus. This substance also augments the amount of acetylcholine released from nerve terminals in the hippocampus and acts similarly on GABA release in the cortex. In addition to these effects in transmitter production and release, alpha-GPC facilitates the responses on neurons to their appropriate transmitters and thereby enhances communication between brain cells.

How has it been tested? What are the risks, if any?

Alpha-GPC has been tested in rats and in several papers consistently found to facilitate learning of avoidance tasks and to counteract the amnesia-producing effects of drugs that reduce the concentration of acetylcholine in the brain. The testing of alpha-GPC in humans is much more limited. There have been two open trials in which alpha-GPC was beneficial to the memory and attentional functioning of patients with cognitive impairments due to circulatory problems. There was one double-blind placebo-controlled trial in which this drug was similarly effective in cognitively impaired people that were probably in the early stages of Alzheimer's disease. There have been no studies of the effects of alpha-GPC in healthy individuals.

Significant side effects of using alpha-GPC have not been reported. The most frequent complaints were heartburn, nausea, insomnia, and headache, each occurring in less than 1 percent of patients.

Typical dosages

One gram (1,000 mg) to 1,200 mg per day was used in the clinical trials in people.

Contraindications

There are no known contraindications for the use of alpha-GPC.

The plain facts

Alpha-GPC appears to be a safe drug that preliminary studies suggest may be of benefit in enhancing the cognitive abilities of people in the early stages of cognitive deterioration due to circulatory problems or Alzheimer's disease. In contrast, there is no evidence that alpha-GPC would be of any help to healthy people. If, as several have suggested, the effectiveness of this drug depends on its ability to increase acetylcholine levels in the brain, it is doubtful that alpha-GPC would be of much use to normal people since acetylcholine levels are typically adequate unless there is illness.

Benefits: 2
Risks: 1

ANIRACETAM
Prescription drug; available through Internet suppliers

What is it?

Aniracetam is structurally related to the first smart drug, piracetam, and is a member of a larger group of similarly acting drugs called the racetams.

Its reputation

Aniracetam is hyped as a more powerful cousin of piracetam with similar though stronger beneficial effects on memory and without significant side effects.

The drug's effect on the brain

As with all of the members of the racetam group, little is known of this drug's mechanisms of action in the brain. There are, however, a few studies available and these suggest potentially interesting effects. Certain types of brain damage in rats cause a decrease in brain metabolism. Aniracetam helps maintain normal levels of brain metabolism in the presence of this brain injury. Aniracetam also has beneficial effects during ischemia. During brain ischemia, the condition characterized by abnormally decreased blood flow to the brain, damage to neurons is caused by the production of toxic free radicals. Aniracetam decreases the free radical formation during brain ischemia. Aniracetam also has effects on certain types of receptor for the neurotransmitter glutamate. Glutamate is found throughout the brain, where it acts as an excitatory transmitter. Among its many functions in the brain, many scientists believe that glutamate is important for the formation of memory. While aniracetam probably has effects on certain glutamate receptors, it is not yet known if these effects would help, hinder, or have no effect on the formation of memory.

How has it been tested? What are the risks, if any?
There has been extensive testing in laboratory animals, primarily rats, and aniracetam consistently improves learning in a variety of tasks and restores the learning ability of older rats.

The testing has been much less extensive in people and the results are promising though mixed. In double-blind placebo-controlled studies of patients with Alzheimer's, one trial showed a beneficial effect on cognitive functioning, particularly memory, while the second showed no positive influence of the drug. This discrepancy may be due to differences in the types of patients included in the trials. The first study was careful to use patients with early Alzheimer's while the second may have included more advanced patients who had deteriorated further and were more difficult to treat. A third trial, using patients suffering from dementia due to decreased circulation, also showed a positive effect of aniracetam on memory. Unfortunately this study was not double-blind.

Research on aniracetam's effects on the brain showed that this drug was a free radical scavenger and, as such, might be helpful in conditions in which the brain's oxygen supply was decreased. A double-blind placebo-controlled study investigated this in ten healthy young adults by assessing their neuropsychological functioning under normal conditions and after they had been made temporarily hypoxic. During hypoxia, performance deteriorated on tests of attention and memory. However, in the presence of aniracetam, the study subjects performed normally despite hypoxia.

The hype concerning aniracetam's safety appears to be true; none of the trials reported significant side effects. Caution is still needed since there have been relatively few studies of aniracetam in people, so that significant risks have not been ruled out.

Typical dosages
One to 1.5 grams per day were used in the clinical trials. However, the metabolism of aniracetam in older individuals is four to seven times slower than in young adults. Although overdose effects have not been described, caution should be shown by older people since the drug will remain in their body for a longer period.

Contraindications
There are no known contraindications.

The plain facts
Aniracetam appears to be a safe drug with hints of beneficial effects on memory functioning in people in the early stages of

senility. In addition, there are also suggestions that aniracetam may protect the brain against the effects of lack of oxygen. Unfortunately there is no information concerning aniracetam's possible benefits for healthy young to middle-aged adults.

Benefits: 2½
Risks: ½

BACOPA
Herb; available through Internet suppliers

What is it?
Bacopa, short for *Bacopa monnieri,* is a plant that grows in the water along the banks of lakes and rivers and is also known as water hyssop. The herbal medicine derived from this plant is also referred to as brahmi, its name in Sanskrit. Originally from India, bacopa is now also found in several Florida regions.

Its reputation
Bacopa is reputed to have been used in traditional medicine in India for at least hundreds of years. It is also used extensively in China, Cuba, and Indonesia. It reportedly improves mental clarity and is thought to be useful in the treatment of memory problems, anxiety, epilepsy, schizophrenia, arthritis, asthma, bronchitis, hair loss, and water retention.

The drug's effect on the brain
The effects of bacopa on the brain are a mystery; there are no reports in any mainstream medical or scientific journals concerning the effects of this substance on the central nervous sys-

tem. Indeed, a review of the available scientific literature revealed only two papers describing any effects of bacopa on the body. The first indicated that bacopa has antioxidant properties and the second that this compound can act as a calcium channel blocker.

How has it been tested? What are the risks, if any?

There have been no trials published in any mainstream medical or scientific journals, either double-blind, single-blind, or open, concerning the effects of bacopa on any aspect of cognitive functioning in people. There is a report that this herb makes it easier for rats to learn to avoid painful shocks, though whether this influence was specifically on learning or if there is any relevance to people is entirely unknown.

Typical dosages

Typical doses cannot be specified. There appear to be at least two active ingredients in bacopa, bacosides A and B, and different commercially available preparations do not state the concentrations of these constituents.

Contraindications

There are no known contraindications.

The plain facts

If you would prefer to take a drug of unproven effectiveness and with unknown actions in the body, a drug whose risks are unclear and whose contraindications are similarly murky, bacopa is made to order. If, however, your decision of whether or not to put a substance into your body is based on a logical weighing of potential benefits against potential risks, you are advised to steer clear.

Benefits: 0

Risks: 4

CAFFEINE

What is it?

Caffeine is derived from a variety of plants that grow all over the world. It is believed that the stimulating properties of these plants were discovered thousands of years ago and that paleolithic man was perhaps the first to make beverages from the leaves of caffeine-containing plants.

Its reputation

Caffeine is thought to be a mild stimulant that counteracts fatigue and that increases mental alertness. Too much caffeine is commonly believed to lead to feelings of anxiety, cause upset stomach, and to disrupt activities that require precise movements, particularly of the fingers (i.e., fine motor control).

The drug's effect on the brain

Although caffeine has many effects on the physiology of living cells, the action that seems to be most relevant to its behavioral properties is its antagonism of adenosine. Adenosine is a neurotransmitter that is released by brain cells, some of which inhibit the activity of other neurons that release dopamine. By blocking adenosine's actions, caffeine enhances the release of dopamine in the brain. Dopamine is involved in many behavioral activities; those that appear most relevant to the actions of caffeine are activation, control of movement, and the subjective experience of pleasure.

How has it been tested? What are the risks, if any?
Caffeine has been more extensively tested, on healthy people, than any other drug discussed in this book. The results have been amazingly consistent whether the trial was open, single-blind, or double-blind. Caffeine has little or no effect on cognitive processes such as memory and executive functioning but increases alertness, improves reaction time, and facilitates the ability to process information. With increasing doses, the fine motor abilities of some people become less efficient and precise.

Caffeine, with moderate use, is quite safe. A fatal dose would be reached by consuming forty cups of strong coffee within a short time period. Excessive use can cause upset stomach, increased urination, jitteriness, and disruption of sleep. Although there have been suggestions that caffeine could cause certain cancers, heart disease, trigger cardiac arrthymias, decrease fertility, increase fibrocystic breast disease, and cause osteoporosis, the weight of current research indicates that these fears are unfounded. The elevation in blood pressure caused by caffeine is mild, short-lived, and less than that associated with normal activities of daily living. Some people complain that they are "addicted" to caffeine. Some people who consume caffeine on a daily basis do experience mild withdrawal symptoms (e.g., headache) upon cessation of use.

Typical dosages
Caffeine is not only present in many beverages in addition to coffee and tea but is also found in many soft drinks and in chocolate. Two cups of coffee or tea, or about twenty ounces of caffeinated soft drink per day is safe for most people.

Contraindications
Due to caffeine's diuretic effects, people with kidney disease should consult their physicians.

The plain facts
Caffeine is a mild stimulant, that with moderate use, is quite safe. Its advertised ability to increase mental alertness has been confirmed in numerous studies.

Benefits: 2
Risks: ½

CENTROPHENOXINE
Nonprescription drug; available through Internet suppliers

What is it?
Centrophenoxine, also commonly known and sold as Lucidril, is a nootropic principally composed of DMAE (see entry on DMAE in this chapter) and another compound that is similar to auxins (plant hormones).

Its reputation
Centrophenoxine is reputed to be an antiaging drug that enhances memory and boosts mental energy levels.

The drug's effect on the brain
Centrophenoxine has a number of interesting effects in the brain that suggest that its use should be investigated in people. It has been shown to be a strong antioxidant and free radical scavenger and so might be useful in counteracting what are perhaps the main causes of age-related deteriora-

tion in brain cell activity. Tests of centrophenoxine's ability to halt some signs of age-related brain deterioration has been confirmed, at least in laboratory animals. A number of changes occur in the brains of experimental animals that are similar to what happens in humans. Lipofuscin, the "aging" pigment, increasingly accumulates in neurons as we get older. The number of synapses, the basis for information transfer between neurons, also decreases with age, as the ability to learn certain types of information deteriorates. In some studies, centrophenoxine prevented these age-related changes in rats, while in other studies, no such effects were observed.

How has it been tested? What are the risks, if any?
Unfortunately there have not been many tests of centrophenoxine's efficacy in people and, of the few existing trials, only two are methodologically sound enough to warrant discussion. In one double-blind placebo-controlled trial, centrophenoxine improved memory performance in moderately demented people. A similar study, using healthy elderly people with mild cognitive difficulties, also showed that centrophenoxine enhanced memory ability.

In general, the risks of centrophenoxine use appear to be minimal, with only stomachache and jitteriness seen in a minority of users. There is one disquieting report, however, that this drug caused seizures in a few patients. Unfortunately it was not clear if these people, who all had cerebrovascular insufficiency, were already suffering a seizure disorder and that drug use caused an exacerbation, or if centrophenoxine triggered convulsions in patients who had never had such an experience.

The uncertainty concerning the seizure potential of centrophenoxine illustrates the potential problems in using a drug that has not been extensively tested. The aforementioned trial of centrophenoxine's effects in moderately demented people exposed only twenty-five patients to the drug. If an adverse effect is seen in only one in a hundred patients, it is likely that such a small trial would not detect it. However, the likelihood that one out of a hundred people taking a drug will have a serious side effect, such as convulsions, is an unacceptably high risk.

Typical dosages
Smart drug advocates suggest doses from 1 to 3 grams daily.

Contraindications
Due to the possible risk of convulsions, centrophenoxine is contraindicated for people with epilepsy and other seizure disorders. In addition, it should be avoided by people with high blood pressure.

The plain facts
Centrophenoxine has a number of effects that suggest it has potential for beneficial effects on cognitive functioning in people. Preliminary results from trials testing its efficacy in people show that this drug is promising for both for healthy people and those in the early stages of senility. Unfortunately more work is needed not only to definitively establish this drug's effectiveness but also to determine its risks.

Benefits: 1
Risks: 4

CHOLINE, LECITHIN, PHOSPHATIDYLCHOLINE
Dietary supplement; available over the counter

What is it?

Choline is a precursor of the acetylcholine, found in high concentrations throughout the brain. In other words, the brain uses choline as one of the building blocks when it is producing more acetylcholine. Choline is found in the dietary supplement lecithin in the form of choline and its close relative phosphatidylcholine. Lecithin is present in many foods such as egg yolks and soybeans and is also used as a thickener in foods such as ice cream and margarine.

Its reputation

Choline, lecithin, and phosphatidylcholine are advertised as dietary supplements that will improve memory abilities. These claims are based upon research findings from the laboratory and from the clinic. In early laboratory research, acetylcholine received a great deal of attention as a transmitter that was especially important for learning and memory. Subsequently it was also shown that in Alzheimer's disease, an early symptom of which is memory loss, the concentrations of acetylcholine in the brain drop dramatically. Because of these facts, some have suggested that memory could be improved, not only in Alzheimer's sufferers but also in healthy people with memory problems, by increasing their brain levels of acetylcholine by supplementation with choline, lecithin, or phosphatidylcholine.

The drug's effect on the brain

The rationale for using these substances is to provide the brain with what it needs to produce acetylcholine, in the expectation that the brain's concentrations of this transmitter will increase. Unfortunately, this is not what happens when a healthy person performs dietary supplementation with choline, lecithin, or phosphatidylcholine. The ability of these compounds to gain access to the brain, through the blood-brain barrier (BBB—explained in Chapter 3), is very precisely regulated. Unless there is a shortage of acetylcholine in the brain, the high levels of precursor circulating in the blood are not allowed to pass through the BBB.

Acetylcholine deficiencies can be caused by certain diseases or as the result of increased activity of neurons that use this neurotransmitter. However, it should be recognized that for neuronal activity-related decreases of acetylcholine, the level of precursors found in a normal diet provide more than enough to supply the brain with sufficient acetylcholine; dietary supplementation is superfluous.

How has it been tested? What are the risks, if any?
Cholinergic precursors have been tested, primarily in double-blind placebo-controlled trials, with mixed results in both normal persons and in Alzheimer's patients. Augmentation of memory was seen in one study of normal persons while no effect was observed in three other studies. Similarly, improvements in memory were seen in one study of Alzheimer's patients and no effect in three additional trials. Neither the scientific rigor nor the size of the drug dose differentiated the research in which beneficial effects were found from those trials in which no effects were observed.

Cholinergic precursors, either lecithin or phosphatidylcholine, have also been tested in combination with other drugs in attempting to treat Alzheimer's disease. A double-blind placebo-controlled trial of phosphatidylcholine used with the smart drug piracetam (discussed at length elsewhere in this chapter) showed no benefits. In contrast, combination of acetylcholine precursors with drugs that prevent the breakdown of newly synthesized acetylcholine, so called acetylcholinesterase inhibitors (e.g., tacrine hydrochloride, sold as Cognex, and physostigmine), had more optimistic results. Two of three double-blind placebo-controlled studies showed beneficial effects on cognitive status in Alzheimer's patients.

The risks of choline and related compounds appear to be minimal. Very high doses are associated with gastrointestinal distress, sweating, salivation, and anorexia, symptoms sufficiently unpleasant for most people to prevent repeated use of such high doses.

Typical dosages
Choline has been recommended in doses as high as 3 grams per day in three divided doses. Because lecithin is not pure choline, higher doses are suggested by commercial suppliers.

Contraindications
There is no clear or definitive scientific evidence of any contraindications for the use of choline, lecithin, or phosphatidylcholine.

The plain facts
There is weak scientific evidence that choline, lecithin, or phosphatidylcholine might have mild beneficial effects on memory in either healthy people or Alzheimer's patients. In contrast, there is stronger evidence for the positive actions of these compounds for treating Alzheimer's disease when used in combination with acetylcholinesterase inhibitors. It should be noted that the latter class of drugs has a number of side

effects, contraindications, and risks and therefore should only be taken under the close supervision of a physician. However, it is unlikely that normal people with memory problems would profit from drugs designed to treat brain abnormalities caused by Alzheimer's disease for reasons that are discussed in Chapter 1.

Benefits: ½
Risks: ½

CITICOLINE
Nonprescription drug; available through Internet suppliers

What is it?
Cytidine 5´-diphosphocholine, CDP-choline, or citicoline is a compound that is involved in the production of essential elements of cell membranes and is a precursor to phosphatidylcholine (see entry on choline).

Its reputation
Citicoline is advertised as the "most effective choline to improve mental function and repair neurological dysfunction."[*]

The drug's effect on the brain
Citicoline is used in the brain to synthesize important constituents of neuronal cell membranes. It is thought that this function of citicoline is involved in brain cell maintenance and repair after injury. Citicoline also increases energy metabolism in the brain and increases the concentrations of the neurotransmitters norepinephrine and dopamine. Re-

---

[*]http://www.lifeextensionvitamins.com/lifeextensionvitamins/cdcholinecaps.html

search using laboratory animals shows that this substance protects brain cells from damage due to oxygen deprivation and improves learning and memory in aging. In addition, citicoline lessens the traumatic effects of head trauma in rats, reducing edema and limiting neuronal damage.

How has it been tested? What are the risks, if any?
Although this drug has received very limited testing, the sparse information available is positive. In two open studies with Alzheimer's disease patients, citicoline improved memory attention and general orientation. More convincing was a double-blind placebo-controlled trial in which repeated administration of citicoline improved verbal memory functioning in elderly persons, possibly with early Alzheimer's. A similar finding was obtained in another placebo-controlled trial with elderly people that showed no obvious signs of Alzheimer's disease. In confirmation of the studies using laboratory animals, citicoline, administered in a double-blind placebo-controlled trial to persons who had suffered traumatic brain injury, promoted recovery of cognitive impairment. In another study, however, citicoline did not improve neurological functioning in stroke patients.

Serious risks of citicoline treatment have not been identified. The most common side effect, observed in about 4 percent of people, was gastrointestinal distress. Other adverse reactions included decreases in blood pressure and mild drops in white blood cell counts.

Typical dosages
In the research studies in which citicoline improved memory functioning, these positive effects were observed with daily doses of 300–1,000 mg.

Contraindications

In view of citicoline's possible effects on white blood cell counts, patients who are immunocompromised, either through disease or medication (e.g., organ transplant patients, patients receiving corticosteroids), should consult their physician before taking this drug. Similarly, persons with low blood pressure or those taking medications for high blood pressure (e.g., beta blockers) should also consult their physician before taking this drug.

The plain facts

Although not extensively tested, there is consistent evidence that citicoline has beneficial effects on memory in elderly persons and in Alzheimer's patients. No studies have yet been performed to determine if this drug would be similarly beneficial in younger healthy patients.

Benefits: 3
Risks: 1

DEPRENYL, ELDEPRYL, OR SELEGILINE

Prescription drug; available in pharmacies by prescription and without prescription through Internet suppliers

---

What is it?

Eldepryl, also known as selegiline hydrochloride or deprenyl, is sold in the United States as a prescription drug that is widely used for the treatment of Parkinson's disease.

Its reputation

Advocates of deprenyl use for purposes other than treating Parkinson's disease claim that this drug fights off the effects of aging, not only on the brain but also other organ systems and, in so doing, increases longevity.

The drug's effect on the brain

One of deprenyl's major actions, the one that recommends its use in Parkinson's disease, is to increase the actions of dopamine in the brain. It accomplishes this not by stimulating the production of dopamine, increasing its release, or by stimulating its receptors. Rather, deprenyl inhibits the actions of enzymes that metabolize (break down) dopamine. In addition, there is evidence that suggests but does not conclusively demonstrate that also deprenyl acts as an antioxidant, free radical scavenger, and neuroprotective agent in the brain.

How has it been tested? What are the risks, if any?

Deprenyl has been extensively tested for efficacy in Alzheimer's disease in double-blind placebo-controlled trials. For the most part, the effects of deprenyl were beneficial though exceedingly mild and not clearly exerted upon specific cognitive processes (e.g., memory, attention). The most thorough of the trials reported positive influences on patients' ability to perform their routine activities of daily living or on general measures of disorientation, but only mild or no changes at all on specific tests of memory, attention, or cognitive functioning. The bottom line concerning its effectiveness with Alzheimer's disease is that despite the potential for enormous profits if deprenyl could be marketed as a treatment for Alzheimer's disease, no drug company has done so.

Deprenyl has also been tested for possible beneficial cognitive effects in patients with other disorders. Many patients with Parkinson's disease experience cognitive difficulties in addition to their problems with movement. Deprenyl, in double-blind placebo-controlled trials, was without positive effect in patients with early Parkinson's disease.

There appear to be few studies of deprenyl's effects in healthy people; a MEDLINE search turned up only one trial that assessed effects on cognition. In this study, deprenyl was mildly depressant, slowed reaction time, and decreased the speed at which the brain processed information. Unfortunately no objective and methodologically sound trials of deprenyl's effects on memory or attentional functioning in healthy young, middle-aged, or elderly people could be found.

Deprenyl's potential to increase longevity has been tested in studies involving a variety of animals and in the majority, drug treatment appeared to increase life span. So, if you're a beagle, a rat, or a fruit fly, you'd probably want to consider taking deprenyl. But what if you're a person? Unfortunately the data concerning deprenyl's effects on life span in humans is sparse and certainly does not suggest that it increases longevity. Indeed, several trials in which the long-term effects of deprenyl were measured in Parkinson's patients suggests that, if anything, mortality might be increased. In addition, one large study suggests the death rate is higher in persons who are taking deprenyl even if they are not Parkinson's patients. It should be pointed out that the issue has not yet been resolved and that there is no consensus that deprenyl increases mortality. However, there is not even a hint that deprenyl will allow you to live longer.

Fairly common side effects of deprenyl include nausea, dizziness, and stomach pain. There also are a variety of risks associated with deprenyl use in certain circumstances. Deprenyl can result in postural hypotension, a significant lowering of blood pressure when you rise from a prone position so severe as to result in a loss of equilibrium and a fall. It should be noted that injury from falls due to this adverse effect has been hypothesized as the reason that the death rate may be elevated in deprenyl users.

It is unclear the extent to which risk is attached to the breakdown products of deprenyl's metabolism (i.e., the chemicals that are produced when the body inactivates deprenyl). Metabolism of deprenyl produces, among other compounds, amphetamine and methamphetamine. Several investigators have suggested that the concentrations of these neurotoxic substances are too low to be of concern. However, the lowest concentrations of amphetamine and methamphetamine that are toxic, when these drugs are present constantly as is the case when deprenyl is taken, is not known. The fact that deprenyl can cause rapid heart rate, insomnia, and hallucinations, common side effects of amphetamine and methamphetamine, indicates that the low concentrations of these compounds are probably high enough to have adverse biological effects.

In addition to the preceding there are also serious and potentially fatal risks associated with using an excessive dose of deprenyl. Overdose can occur either when the recommended maximum daily dose of 10 mg is exceeded or by interaction with estrogens and progesterone typically present in birth control pills. Concomitant use of oral contraceptives can cause a twentyfold increase in the amount of deprenyl that reaches your brain. Deprenyl, when used in the appropriate low concentrations, has a specific action that slows down the metabolism of dopamine. At high concentrations, such as occurs when taking more than 10 mg per day or due to interactions with oral contraceptives, deprenyl has more general effects and such ordinarily benign activities as eating cheese or other tyramine-containing foods or drinking a single glass of wine can result in hypertensive reactions and even be fatal.

Typical dosages

Under no circumstances should a dose of 10 mg per day be exceeded. Oral contraceptives greatly enhance the effects of deprenyl so that an ordinarily safe dose can lead to life-threatening complications.

Contraindications

In addition to the interactions with oral contraceptives, deprenyl in combination with either opioids such as Demerol, tricyclic antidepressants, or serotonin-reuptake inhibitors such as Prozac is potentially fatal.

The plain facts

Despite rave notices, deprenyl has little to recommend its use for cognitive enhancement in people with Alzheimer's disease and even less to recommend its use in healthy people. In addition, while deprenyl may increase life span in dogs, rats, and flies, there is no indication that it does so in people. If you find deprenyl's antioxidant and free radical scavenging properties attractive, there are other substances available with similar actions that are much safer to use.

Benefits: 1
Risks: 4

DILANTIN
Prescription drug; available by prescription in pharmacies and without prescription through Internet suppliers

What is it?
Dilantin, also known by the generic name phenytoin, was introduced into general use in 1938 as an anticonvulsant, a drug that is used to prevent the seizures of epilepsy.

Its reputation
A variety of sources claim that Dilantin, in addition to its beneficial influences on epilepsy, also is a potent cognitive aid. Used in normal people, this drug is said to improve concentration and general cognitive functioning, particularly in the elderly, and even to increase IQ. Although it is recognized that there is a possibility of side effects with Dilantin, such adverse events are said to be relatively uncommon and the drug claimed to be fairly safe.

The drug's effect on the brain
Dilantin's anticonvulsant actions stem from its ability to affect the basic processes that occur when a neuron becomes activated. Prior to activation, during the so-called resting state, there is a high concentration of sodium and calcium immediately surrounding the neuron and a high concentration inside. The first event during activation is a rapid flow of sodium, and sometimes calcium, into the neuron through sodium channels, followed by a rapid flow of potassium out of the neuron. The resting state is restored when the potassium streams back into the brain cell followed by the egress of sodium. Dilantin acts by curtailing the flow of sodium, potassium, and possibly calcium, thereby rendering the neuron less

excitable and less likely to be available for activation under conditions that would ordinarily result in a seizure. In the presence of Dilantin, brain cells are more difficult to activate and less likely to fire rapidly and repetitively. These changes in a neuron's excitability are essential for the prevention of seizures but are they likely to improve the brain's ability to control cognitive processes?

How has it been tested? What are the risks, if any?
One of the earliest papers suggesting a beneficial effect of Dilantin on cognitive processing was a double-blind placebo-controlled trial involving ten elderly subjects, in which intellectual abilities were measured by repeated applications of an intelligence test. The authors felt that the drug treatment increased IQ, improved long-term memory and social comprehension, increased visuomotor coordination, and enhanced the ability to learn new information. Unfortunately, there are a number of serious shortcomings in this study that render its results difficult to take seriously. Too few people were tested, IQ tests were administered three times within six weeks (a procedure that results in spuriously inflated scores), and the meaning of scores on specific parts of the IQ tests were most probably misinterpreted. Two more recent studies, using much larger numbers of subjects and better methods, examined the performance on IQ tests of children taking Dilantin. In both studies, Dilantin-exposed children had significantly lower IQs. Although it is possible that Dilantin's effects on the intellectual functioning of the elderly (first study) differ from those in children (second and third studies), numerous trials in recent years assessing influences on the cognitive abilities of adults indicate that, at best, the drug has no effect, and, more frequently, is disruptive.

Thus, the benefit half of the risk/benefit ratio is hardly encouraging—but what about the risks? Unfortunately, the list of possible side effects is so extensive that what follows can only be considered an overview. The most typical side effects are due to Dilantin's actions on the brain and include slurred speech, balance problems, nystagmus (involuntary rapid and repetitive movement of the eyes), mental confusion, dizziness, headaches, insomnia, and twitching. Emergence of a skin rash is one of the first signs of toxicity and an indication for immediate termination of drug administration. Dilantin can induce a variety of skin disorders that are serious and can be fatal, including toxic epidermal necrolysis, lupus erythematosus, and purpuric dermatitis. Other adverse reactions due to Dilantin are hyperglycemia, osteomalacia, toxic hepatitis, and liver damage. Serious and sometimes fatal blood disorders include agranulocytosis, thrombocytopenia, and leukopenia, coarsening of facial skin, overgrowth of the lips, gums, and tissue lining the mouth, and Peyronie's disease. Since Dilantin also inhibits thyroid function, supplemental thyroid hormone may be necessary. Dilantin may also interfere with the availability of certain vitamins, thereby necessitating supplementation.

Dilantin is broken down in the liver so that people with liver dysfunction are more likely to develop symptoms of toxicity at lower doses. Even in healthy people, however, there is a great deal of variability from person to person in the dosage level of Dilantin that is therapeutic as compared to the dose that is toxic. When Dilantin is used as a treatment for seizures, the circulating drug levels are typically monitored very closely via weekly blood tests.

Dilantin interacts with a variety of other drugs. The following list should not be considered to be comprehensive:

alcohol, amiodarone, chloramphenicol, chlordiazepoxide, diazepam (Valium), disulfram, dicumarol, estrogens (some birth control pills), H-2 antagonists, isoniazid, methylphenidate (Ritalin), phenothiazines (some antipsychotic drugs), phenylbutazone, salicylates (including aspirin), succinimides, sulfonamides, tolbutamide, and trazadone. Dilantin also lowers the effectiveness of many drugs including corticosteroids, Coumadin and similar anticoagulants, digoxin, deoxycycline, estrogens, furosemide, quinidine, rifampin, theophylline, and vitamin D. For a more extensive index of drug interactions and side effects, consult the current *Physicians' Desk Reference*.

Typical dosages

This can best be determined by a physician using blood tests to monitor circulating drug levels.

Contraindications

It is our opinion that Dilantin is contraindicated for everyone other than those for whom this drug is prescribed by their physician.

The plain facts

The scientific literature does not support claims that Dilantin has beneficial effects on cognitive functioning. In addition, there are so many possible side effects and potential drug interactions that use of this drug without medical supervision is dangerous. In short, there is no reason for a healthy person to take Dilantin and many reasons to avoid it.

Benefits: 0
Risks: 5

DMAE

Dietary supplement; available over the counter and through Internet suppliers

What is it?

Dimethylaminoethanol (DMAE), also sold as the related compound deanol, is a precursor of choline and is found in trace concentrations in the brain as well as in various foods, particularly seafood.

Its reputation

DMAE is thought, by some, to be converted in the body to choline, which, in turn, is converted to acetylcholine in the brain. It is sold as a memory enhancer, a mild stimulant, and also as a general "antiaging" drug.

The drug's effect on the brain

DMAE does indeed lead to increased choline levels in the brain but, unless there is a deficiency, the final step of conversion to acetylcholine does not occur. Thus, unless there is a condition that leads to deficiency of acetylcholine, a problem not present in healthy people, DMAE does not increase acetylcholine levels in the brain. The claims of DMAE's antiaging effects also do not hold up to experimental scrutiny, at least when tested in lab animals. Cherkin and Exkardt found that Japanese quail treated with DMAE had a shorter life span than control animals. In addition, DMAE also did not lessen the impact of aging on these animals' sexual behavior or learning ability.

In contrast to the disappointing evidence concerning DMAE's effects on acetylcholine and aging, other studies show that this drug has neuroprotective effects. DMAE treatment protects brain cells from damage due to hypoxia.

Although the mechanism of this neuroprotection is not known, other work has shown that DMAE is an effective scavenger of free radicals.

How has it been tested? What are the risks, if any?

The effects of DMAE in people has not been systematically tested using objective scientific methods. Although tested on patients with Alzheimer's disease, the majority of clinical trials were open studies; only one double-blind placebo-controlled trial was found. However, whether the trial was open or double-blind, DMAE was shown to have a similar lack of efficacy. A review of the biomedical literature revealed no acceptable studies of DMAE's effects in healthy people. Interestingly, in a double-blind placebo-controlled trial, DMAE was found to enhance cognitive functioning in children with "minimal brain dysfunction" (probably ADHD).

There is little in the published reports to suggest that there are serious side effects of DMAE use. Overdosage can result in headaches, muscle tension, and insomnia. DMAE should not be used by people with bipolar disorder, and people with epilepsy should be closely monitored by a physician.

Typical dosages

Dosages ranged from 500 mg to 1,800 mg per day in the clinical trials.

Contraindications

As discussed, DMAE is contraindicated for persons with bipolar disorder.

The plain facts

Although DMAE appears to be relatively safe, the few clinical trials that could be reviewed do not provide evidence that it would be effective in persons with Alzheimer's disease or other forms of senility. There is simply no reliable data pertaining to its possible uses in healthy people, and experimental studies do not strongly suggest that DMAE would be particularly useful in fighting off the effects of growing older.

Benefits: ½
Risks: 3

FIPEXIDE
Nonprescription drug; available through Internet suppliers

What is it?
Fipexide (also known as Attentil, BP662, and Visilor) is a mild stimulant whose mechanisms of action are unclear.

Its reputation
Fipexide is a stimulant that is claimed to lack the side effects of amphetamine and to act as an enhancer of cognitive processes in general and learning in particular. Several advocates of fipexide suggest that this drug's effects are mediated by its ability to increase dopamine levels in the brain.

The drug's effect on the brain
Fipexide appears to facilitate the actions of dopamine, although it does so indirectly and not by increasing the levels of this neurotransmitter in the brain. Neurons that release dopamine are inhibited by the actions of enkephalins, another class of neurotransmitters that are the brain's own morphine-like substances. It is thought that fipexide inhibits synaptic transmission mediated by enkephalins and, in so

doing, releases dopamine neurons from inhibition so that they can fire more frequently and release more dopamine.

How has it been tested? What are the risks, if any?

An exhaustive search through the biomedical literature turned up only one clinical trial of fipexide's efficacy in people. This double-blind placebo-controlled study tested the cognitive abilities of elderly people with moderate to severe cognitive problems possibly due to Alzheimer's disease and other forms of senility. Fipexide had statistically significant beneficial effects on memory, attention, and mood. Unfortunately, there seems to have been no attempt to repeat this trial nor have there been any tests of this drug's effects in healthy people. However, consideration of the risks of fipexide use may indicate the reason for this lack of follow-up.

According to published reports, fipexide carries a risk of liver damage so significant as to require organ transplant. In addition, fipexide also induces high fever often associated with eosinophilia (an increase in the number of eosinophils, a type of white blood cell, circulating in the blood, a condition associated with allergies or inflammation).

Typical dosages

In the lone published clinical trial, 600 mg per day was administered.

Contraindications

Based on its effects on the liver, fipexide is contraindicated in persons with hepatitis and other forms of liver disorder. If fipexide is actually a stimulant, this compound is likely contraindicated for persons with anxiety disorders and those suffering from insomnia. It is also possible, in view of fipexide's advertised stimulant properties, that there may be some risk for people with heart problems.

The plain facts
Although there is one promising study in persons with Alzheimer's disease, there is too little information to determine if fipexide has real benefits for people. In addition, what little is known strongly suggests that the potential side effects of fipexide are very serious and that its use is ill advised.

Benefits: ½
Risks: 5

GEROVITAL
Nonprescription drug; available through Internet suppliers

What is it?
Gerovital, also known as GH-3, is primarily the local anesthetic procaine with the addition of an antioxidant and a preservative.

Its reputation
Gerovital is touted as an antiaging formulation that fights off the deleterious effects of age on cognition as well as on the body's other organ systems. One Internet source suggests that gerovital is beneficial in arthritis, migraine, both high and low blood pressure, Parkinson's disease, multiple sclerosis, herpes, impotence, balding, heart disease, poor eyesight, and several other conditions. It states that this compound "... has been established as possibly the most exciting medical discov-

ery for mankind since the principles of medical hygiene were reluctantly accepted by the profession in the 19th century."*

The drug's effect on the brain
Gerovital inhibits the actions of an enzyme in the brain called monoamine oxidase (MAO). MAO breaks down the neurotransmitters epinephrine, norepinephrine, dopamine, and serotonin, an important function that in the healthy person maintains transmitter levels at appropriate concentrations. In certain diseases, e.g., Parkinson's, wherein dopamine levels decrease, or depression in which serotonin levels are thought to decrease, MAO inhibitors sometimes can be of some use by elevating transmitter levels.

How has it been tested? What are the risks, if any?
There have been numerous testimonials and letters to the editors of various journals describing the potent beneficial influences of gerovital on the degenerative effects of aging. How has gerovital fared in more objective scientific assessments? In reviewing "data from 285 articles and books, describing treatment in 100,000 patients in the past 25 years," A. Ostfield et al. stated: "Except for a possible antidepressant effect, there is no convincing evidence that procaine (or gerovital, of which procaine is the major component) has any value in the treatment of disease in older patients."* More recent double-blind placebo-controlled studies confirmed gerovital's lack of efficacy with psychological or physiological

---

*Gerovital Direct: http://www.sh3.uk/about_gerovital.html

*Ostfield, A., C. M. Smith, and B. A. Stotsky. "The Systemic Use of Procaine in the Treatment of the Elderly: A Review." *Journal of the American Geriatric Society* 25:1–19, 1977.

dysfunctions and further indicated that this formulation also lacked antidepressant effects.

The potential risks of gerovital use are high. Excessive use can result in a variety of symptoms related to brain dysfunction such as tremors, unconsciousness, convulsions, and respiratory arrest. Effects on the cardiovascular system can include low or high blood pressure, slowing of heart rate, and cardiac arrest. Hypersensitivity reactions to the topical use of this drug have been frequently reported.

Typical dosages

Gerovital is administered as either tablets (100 mg/day) or by intramuscular injections (5–10 ml/day, 3 days/week).

Contraindications

Other than patients with hypersensitivity to gerovital, there are no contraindications.

The plain facts

There is no solid evidence that gerovital has beneficial effects on cognitive functioning or that it is an effective antiaging drug. In view of the risks associated with its use, gerovital is not recommended. Although there are many things you can do to slow the aging process and maintain your mental capacities, taking gerovital is not one of them.

Benefits: 0
Risks: 5

GINKGO BILOBA
Herb; available over the counter

What is it?

Ginkgo biloba is a living fossil; it comes from a tree dating back more than 200 million years, which is extinct in the wild but is still flourishing through cultivation for its medicinal purposes. Extracts made from its dried leaves have been used in traditional Chinese medicine for more than 5,000 years for the treatment of, among other things, memory loss. In the last several decades, ginkgo biloba or its extracts have become the most widely used alternative medicine treatment in both Europe (where it is prescribed by physicians) and North America to improve memory functioning in healthy individuals and in persons in the early stages of Alzheimer's disease.

Its reputation

Proponents of ginkgo, particularly those who market it, suggest that its beneficial effects are due to its ability to improve cerebral circulation. If this is actually the case, it is doubtful that this herb would be of much use to anybody other than patients suffering from cerebral atherosclerosis; memory difficulties in healthy individuals are not due to cerebral circulation problems.

The drug's effect on the brain

Ginkgo biloba has been studied by mainstream scientists using traditional, accepted methods for over twenty years and a number of other biological actions have been identified that may have some bearing on its potential for beneficial effects on brain function. There is evidence that, as advertised, this substance does increase cerebral blood flow. In addition, some components of ginkgo extract have strong antioxidant and free radical scavenging qualities and other components of ginkgo extract have potent anti-inflammatory properties.

How has it been tested? What are the risks, if any?
The studies of ginkgo biloba's effects on human memory fall into two groups, those studying Alzheimer's patients and normal individuals. There have been more than fifty trials of ginkgo biloba or its extracts in the treatment of Alzheimer's disease. Close scrutiny reveals that only four of these were sufficiently well designed and controlled to allow a valid evaluation of ginkgo's effects. These four studies showed that ginkgo had a statistically significant (i.e., an effect not due to chance) beneficial effect on Alzheimer's patients' cognitive functioning. The studies that were not included in the group of four lacked placebo control, double-blinding, or objective measurement of cognitive functioning.

In contrast to the numerous studies of ginkgo's effects on Alzheimer's, there have been relatively few evaluations of its effects on normal people. However, like its effects in Alzheimer's patients, it also seems to be beneficial for memory functioning in healthy people. In two double-blind placebo-controlled experiments performed by the same scientist, ginkgo had a positive effect on the memories of healthy female volunteers. Unfortunately, the sample was too small—the effect was shown in fewer than ten individuals— to draw any broad conclusions. In a third such study, performed by a different group of scientists, a ginkgo extract had modest beneficial effects on memory, in contrast to the lack of effect of both the placebo and whole ginkgo biloba. Very recently, ginkgo extract was tested in a much larger number of elderly people. The effects of ginkgo were again positive;

improvement in short-term memory for visual information was seen across the board and memory for verbal information was improved in those people who, before exposure to ginkgo, were most impaired in this area.

The possible basis of ginkgo's beneficial effects bears discussion. Advertisements for ginkgo stress its effect on circulation to the brain as the basis of its positive influences. However, cognitive problems in Alzheimer's disease are due to the death of neurons from structural lesions known as neurofibrillary tangles and neuritic plaques, not from decreased blood flow. In association with these lesions, many neurons are damaged and eventually killed by free radicals, oxidative stress, and inflammation. These processes also play an important toxic role in other dementias of old age. Since ginkgo is a potent free radical scavenger, antioxidant, and anti-inflammatory agent, these properties might be most important for slowing deterioration rather than effects on circulation. In addition, the cumulative effects of free radicals and oxidative stress are thought, by some, to also have an increasing impact on brain functioning as healthy people age. If this is, in fact, the case, ginkgo's antioxidant, free radical scavenging, and anti-inflammatory properties would also be beneficial to healthy people.

Although the risks associated with using ginkgo biloba appear to be minimal, pronouncements of its absolute safety by commercial suppliers, even at high doses, are incorrect. Ginkgo appears to interfere with coagulation and prolongs the time blood takes to clot. Accordingly, persons with preexisting clotting problems, those taking aspirin or warfarin (Coumadin), or otherwise healthy people taking high doses of ginkgo should be cautious when using this herb.

Typical dosages

Ginkgo biloba, used for medicinal purposes, is an extract of the dried leaf of the ginkgo biloba tree. The extract tested in the scientific studies described in this chapter and that typically sold in health food stores is standardized to contain 24 percent ginkgo-flavone glycosides and 6 percent terpenoids. With such an extract the daily dose is 120 to 240 mg per day. With lower potency extracts, dosages would have to be adjusted upward to compensate.

Contraindications

Due to its effects on blood clotting, ginkgo biloba is contraindicated for persons with clotting disorders, such as hemophilia, as well as persons taking anticoagulants, such as Coumadin. If you must take aspirin on a daily basis, ginkgo probably should be avoided.

The plain facts

In summary, there is strong evidence that ginkgo biloba has beneficial effects on the memory functioning abilities of patients with Alzheimer's disease. In addition, while there have been fewer studies of ginkgo's effects in healthy people, there is also increasing evidence that ginkgo biloba can improve memory functioning in this group. The evidence for using ginkgo biloba as a memory aid must be weighed against this herb's potential to cause problems in blood coagulation.

Benefits: 4
Risks: 2

GINSENG
Herb; available over the counter

What is it?

Ginseng is an herb that is native to China, Korea, Japan, Russia, and some regions in North America. Extracts, typically from the root, have been used in traditional Chinese medicine for centuries (some say thousands of years) as an all-purpose treatment for a wide variety of ailments. There are at least three different types of ginseng: American, Siberian, and Asian.

Its reputation

Ginseng is promoted as an adaptogen, a term with currency among herbalists and perhaps scientists in Russia but without general use or meaning in medicine or science. An adaptogen, illiberally defined, is a cure-all or something that's "good for what ails you." Thus, ginseng is supposed to raise your blood pressure if it's low and lower it if it's high, raise your blood sugar if it's low and lower it if it's high, and so on. In addition, ginseng is purported to help your body ward off the effects of fatigue and stress, improve cardiovascular function, help you to sleep, but, at the same time, give you energy, improve immune function, fight cancer, increase resistance to toxins, cure erectile dysfunction and, well . . . do everything anyone could possibly want except cure baldness. Ginseng's advertised effects on cognition, the only claims that we'll examine in this book, are to improve memory, learning, and attention.

The drug's effect on the brain

Laboratory research indicates that ginseng has several interesting biological effects that are of potential benefit to people. Ginsenoside, one of the active ingredients in ginseng, enhances the production of a variety of trophic factors in the brain. Trophic factors act to help brain cells to protect themselves from some toxins, to repair themselves when damaged, and to grow. In addition, ginseng has been shown to be a very strong antioxidant, an action that would protect against the damaging effects of oxygen free radicals.

How has it been tested? What are the risks, if any?
Numerous well-conducted studies have clearly shown that ginseng facilitates learning of a variety of different types of tasks in mice and rats. In addition, ginseng is also able to counteract the debilitating effects of aging on learning abilities in these species and also to reverse the amnesia-producing effects of drugs that decrease the effects of acetylcholine in the brain.

In contrast to the abundance of research concerning ginseng's effects in rodents, there are surprisingly few controlled investigations of its influences on cognition in people. This lack of information is all the more amazing in view of the widespread use of this herb all over the world. There were only four published papers that could be considered and not one was at all persuasive. The first was published in a Chinese medical journal and claimed that ginseng not only had "anti-senility" effects, but also improved immune function and cardiovascular activity. Unfortunately, only a limited translation was available and it is uncertain if the study was open, single-blind, or double-blind. In addition, there was no indication of how any of ginseng's effects were actually measured or if the effects were statistically significant. The three remaining studies were double-blind and placebo-controlled. One found no beneficial effect of ginseng in elderly healthy people but failed to use adequate testing to evaluate cognition. Conversely, a second study did find very strong beneficial effects in a large number of healthy people but, like the preceding trial, also used inadequate testing to evaluate cognitive effects. The sole study in which adequate testing was used found that ginseng had a positive effect on attention and reaction time. Unfortunately, these results must be considered preliminary, as only sixteen people were used as subjects.

There is very little in the existing literature concerning the risks and side effects of ginseng. There have been reports that this herb or its extracts lessens the effects of the blood thinner Coumadin and increases the levels of the heart medication digoxin. Here are the risks of the specific types of ginseng:

American: otherwise safe

Siberian: long-term continuous use not recommended

Asian: nervousness, agitation, and insomnia in some people

Typical dosages

Fifty to 320 mg per day were used in the clinical trials that reported beneficial effects of ginseng. Alternative medicine resources suggest dosages as high as 3,000 mg per day. However, one final point should be considered. There are many different varieties of ginseng grown throughout the world and they differ in their content of the active ingredients, to the extent that they are even known. This problem for the consumer is exacerbated by the lack of standardization in either measuring or reporting on active ingredients.

Contraindications

Dean and Morganthaler indicate that ginseng might be contraindicated for people with hypertension, though the basis for this precaution was not stated. It is also contraindicated in people with heart disease and electrolyte imbalance.

The plain facts

Despite the extravagant claims on the behalf of ginseng's healing powers, there is precious little scientific documentation of its actual effectiveness. Based on laboratory findings concerning its trophic and antioxidant effects as well as its positive influences on learning and memory in rodents, it is plausible that ginseng could be beneficial to people. However plausibility is, unfortunately, not a guarantee of effectiveness. If you choose to use this herb, you must depend primarily on the word of companies whose profit margin rides on whether or not you buy it.

Benefits: 1
Risks: 3

GOTU KOLA
Herb; available over the counter

What is it?

Gotu kola—also known as *Centella asiatica,* Indian pennywort, *Hydrocotyle asiatica,* and talepetrako—is an herb indigenous to countries with hot humid climates (e.g., Africa, India, Sri Lanka, South America, and China) that is promoted as a tonic to increase overall brain function and to improve memory as well as treat virtually every malady known to kill, plague, or annoy humankind.

Its reputation

Gotu kola has been purportedly used widely in Chinese and Indian folk medicine as a stimulant and to promote longevity. According to one Internet source, this herb was consumed by one "professor Li Chung Yon, who reputedly lived 265 years and married 24 times." Whether or not this is a plus depends upon personal taste. It is reported to improve cognitive functioning in general and memory in particular. However, gotu kola is also reported as a cure for uterine cancer, epilepsy, and elephantitis, and is used for the treatment of depression, schizophrenia, congestive heart failure, hepatitis, leprosy, flu, sore throat, low sex drive, and a host of other diseases and unpleasant conditions.

The drug's effect on the brain

We have not been able to find a single study published in a reputable peer-reviewed scientific journal that investigated gotu kola's effects on the brain or behavior in laboratory animals or humans.

How has it been tested? What are the risks, if any?

There have been a few studies of gotu kola's physiological effects indicating that this herb may have important benefits. In one double-blind placebo-controlled study, either 30 mg or 60 mg of gotu kola, administered twice daily for sixty days, improved circulatory functioning without adverse effects. Research using laboratory animals showed that this herb promoted wound healing, retarded the growth of tumors, and enhanced antioxidant activity. There also have been several reports that topical use of gotu kola results in skin rash.

Unfortunately, there have been no scientific studies of gotu kola's effects on cognition, in either humans or laboratory animals. Indeed, there have been no valid investigations of its therapeutic effects in any of the thirty or so diseases for which it is advertised to be effective. As a result of the absence of such work, its risks, side effects, drug interactions, and so on are unknown. However, one of the critical ingredients is thought to be asiaticoside, which can cause sedation in high doses.

Typical dosages

Gotu kola is typically eaten raw in salads, steamed and served with rice, or made into a tea. Since there is little information concerning the identity of its active ingredients, what would constitute an effective dose as compared to an overdose is not known.

Contraindications

Since there are so few studies of gotu kola's effects in people, specific contraindications for its use are not known.

The plain facts

Few if any drugs described in this book match gotu kola for the extravagance of its advertised beneficial effects or for the lack of real evidence to support any of these claims. In addition, little is known concerning its actions in the body or its risk of side effects or drug interactions. What little of this drug's actions (wound healing, pro-antioxidant) have been documented by scientific work indicate that this compound may have health benefits, but the dangers inherent in the lack of information concerning gotu kola's actions result in a decidedly negative risk/benefit ratio.

Benefits: 0
Risks: 4

GUARANA
Herb; available over the counter

What is it?

Guarana, also known as *Paullinia cupana,* is derived from a woody vine that grows in the Brazilian Amazon region. It is advertised as a natural stimulant whose effects on cognition include enhancement of memory and learning.

Its reputation

Guarana is thought to be a caffeine-like compound and is either taken as a capsule or brewed like coffee into a stimulating drink. In addition to uses based upon its advertised activating effects, guarana is also thought to be an aphrodisiac and to be effective for the treatment of headaches, diarrhea, and the symptoms of PMS.

The drug's effect on the brain

There have been no scientific studies of guarana's effects on the brain. Anecdotal reports are fairly consistent in describing stimulating effects similar to those of caffeine, though substantiation in peer-reviewed medical/scientific journals has not yet been published.

How has it been tested? What are the risks, if any?

Two double-blind placebo-controlled trials of guarana's effects in people have been published. The first measured effects on the cognition of healthy elderly people while the second, using similar subjects, assessed not only cognition but also anxiety and sleep. Guarana had no measurable effects in either study. The persuasiveness of these studies is lessened, however, by the fact that caffeine was also tested and found to be without effect. Caffeine has been shown in other scientifically valid studies to have reproducible positive effects on cognition. It is plausible that the tests used to test the efficacy of guarana were not sensitive to its effects.

Although adverse effects of guarana have not been identified in humans, there have been too few studies to support the conclusion that this substance is safe or without side effects. Indeed, it is unlikely that use of guarana is entirely safe since it has been established that guarana inhibits blood platelet aggregation and interferes with blood clotting. A cautionary note was raised in a recent investigation of guarana's cytotoxic (i.e., cell-killing) potential. This research ". . . suggests that the concentration of guarana is of critical importance in its cytotoxic activity and high doses could be harmful to human health." Since there have been no studies that establish guarana's safe and appropriate dose range, there are no guidelines to establish precisely what constitutes a high dose. Other side effects can include nervousness, fast or irregular heartbeat, and upset stomach. Some reports of increased cancer risk have also been made.

Typical doses
Commercially available tablets in the range of 350–500 mg are available with the manufacturer's suggestion of taking 1–2 tablets per day. The basis for this advice is uncertain since no research concerning dosage has been published. This problem is compounded by the fact that analyses of commercially available products showed "that a number of these products may not contain authentic guarana as an active ingredient or contain less than the declared quantity of guarana."

Contraindications

Guarana interferes with blood clotting so that people with clotting disorders such as hemophilia or persons taking blood thinners such as Coumadin or aspirin therapy should avoid this substance. If guarana is actually a stimulant, this compound is likely contraindicated for persons with anxiety disorders and those suffering from insomnia. It is also possible, in view of guarana's advertised stimulant properties, that there may be some risk for people with heart problems.

The plain facts

Although guarana is advertised as a stimulant that can improve cognitive functioning, there is no independent scientific evidence of this compound's stimulating effects, influences on cognition, or effects in the brain. In addition, it is not clear, when guarana is purchased from a commercial supplier, precisely how much of the active ingredient is present or if there's any guarana present at all.

Benefits: 0
Risks: 4

HUPERZINE A

Herb; available over the Internet

What is it?

Huperzine A is derived from *Huperzia serrata,* a moss that grows in China and Hawaii.

Its reputation

Huperzine A is thought to be the active ingredient in the Chinese herbal medicine Qian Ceng Ta and is traditionally used to treat inflammation and fever. Its proponents tout huperzine as a treatment for memory loss in Alzheimer's patients and, in healthy people, as a memory booster as well as a way to enhance concentration ability and energy levels. The source of huperzine's positive effects is thought to reside in its ability to raise the levels of the neurotransmitter acetylcholine in the brain. As mentioned previously (see entry on choline), some researchers believe that acetylcholine is one of the more important neurotransmitters needed for memory formation.

The drug's effect on the brain
The brain very precisely controls its levels of neurotransmitters. When levels decrease, biological signals are given that start the chain of events leading to the synthesis of more transmitter. Conversely, when transmitter levels increase, particularly in synapses, the transmitter is either removed by being transported into axon terminals and/or broken down and inactivated by enzymes designed for that purpose. In the case of the neurotransmitter acetylcholine, the enzymes that break it down are called acetylcholinesterases. Huperzine is a potent acetylcholinesterase inhibitor, an action that allows this compound to increase the brain's acetylcholine levels as advertised.

In addition to its influences on acetylcholine, huperzine also has effects on another neurotransmitter known as glutamate. Glutamate is found throughout the brain where it acts as an excitatory transmitter (see Chapter 3) that, among its many functions, has been specifically implicated in the formation of memory. In addition, during many pathological conditions, glutamate is released from nerve terminals and rises to abnormally high concentrations in the synapse, where it triggers a process called excitotoxicity that ultimately kills brain cells. Huperzine's actions are such that it can facilitate the normal activities of glutamate and block its excitotoxic effects.

How has it been tested? What are the risks, if any?

There have been many tests of huperzine's effects on learning and memory in rats and monkeys. The results consistently show that this drug facilitates learning and memory and can counteract the disruptive effects of experimentally lowering the brain's concentration of acetylcholine. The data pertaining to huperzine's effectiveness in people is much more limited, however. There have been two well-designed double-blind placebo-controlled trials of huperzine's effectiveness with early senility due to Alzheimer's disease and possibly other causes. In both trials huperzine had statistically significant beneficial influences on memory functioning as well general cognitive functioning. Although neither trial mentioned significant side effects, each study used too few subjects (50 and 104) to pronounce the drug as risk free. In addition to these two trials, there apparently have been other trials published in Chinese medical journals that were not available for evaluation.

Typical dosages

The dosages used in the published clinical studies varied from 0.06 to 0.10 mg per day.

Contraindications

There is too little information to determine if there are contraindications.

The plain facts

Whither huperzine? The results from the experiments using animals, although encouraging, are not sufficient to justify huperzine's use by the public. Based on the available published reports, if your pet rat is a slow learner, you might want to consider giving it huperzine. But should you take this drug yourself? Certainly its confirmed biological effects in the brain indicate that, in theory, huperzine might well be beneficial to both Alzheimer's patients and also healthy people with mild memory problems. Unfortunately, there are too few papers published in English that evaluate, using accepted objective methods, huperzine's effectiveness in humans. The fact that there have been so few trials also means that it is difficult to determine the risks or the contraindicated conditions. Until additional work is completed, the best strategy is simply to wait.

Benefits: 2
Risks: 3

HYDERGINE

Prescription drug; also available through Internet suppliers

What is it?

Hydergine is derived from ergot, a parasitic fungus that grows on rye and other grains in Europe and North America. Ergot has been recognized for over two thousand years to be the source of chemicals that could exert powerful and often dangerous effects on the human body. As early as 600 B.C., an Assyrian tablet alluded to a "noxious pustule in the ear of grain"; and in one of the sacred books of the Parsees (400 to

300 B.C.), the following pertinent passage occurs: "Among the evil things created by Angro Maynes are noxious grasses that cause pregnant women to drop the womb and die in childbirth."* In the twentieth century, many interesting drugs have been derived from ergot, including LSD, but also treatments for migraine and Parkinson's disease. Hydergine, also known as ergoloid mesylates, is also a derivative of ergot and was initially targeted toward treating senility.

Its reputation

Hydergine is reputed to be effective in the treatment of senility due to insufficient blood supply to the brain and also to be of use with Alzheimer's patients. Smart drug advocates promote the use of this drug in healthy individuals to increase mental alertness and concentration and to improve memory. The basis of Hydergine's putative beneficial effects is an ability to increase blood flow to the brain, enhance oxygenation, and protect brain cells from the damaging effects of free radicals.

The drug's effect on the brain

In reviewing the existing literature concerning Hydergine's advertised power to augment blood flow to the brain, the 1996 edition of the *Physicians' Desk Reference* concluded that there was not "conclusive evidence that the drug particularly affects cerebral arteriosclerosis or cerebrovascular insufficiency." Although Positron Emission Tomographic (PET) scans in people show that Hydergine does in fact increase

---

*T. W. Rall, "Drugs Affecting Uterine Motility." In *The Pharmacological Basis of Therapeutics*, edited by A. G. Gilman, T. W. Rall, A. S. Nies, and P. Taylor. New York: Pergamon Press, 1990, p. 939.

glucose consumption by brain cells, this finding simply means that the activity of neurons is increased. Such increases do not necessarily indicate beneficial effects as far as cognitive abilities are concerned.

In contrast to the advertised effects on cerebral circulation, Hydergine's free radical scavenging effects were substantiated in the laboratory. In addition, Hydergine was also shown to act as a neuroprotectant in saving brain cells from death due to lack of oxygen.

How has it been tested? What are the risks, if any?
In tests using laboratory animals, Hydergine effectively enhances learning of a variety of different tasks. In people, however, the effects of this drug are by no means as consistent or as encouraging.

A fair number of double-blind placebo-controlled trials that tested Hydergine's beneficial effects on groups of people suffering from either Alzheimer's disease or cerebrovascular insufficiency reported positive results. However, these trials did not use objective tests of cognitive functions that would allow precise judgments about the degree of benefit. Trials that did use such testing either found no benefit of Hydergine or found very modest effects. In reviewing twelve clinical trials up to 1976, it was concluded that "because of the small magnitude of improvement and the absence of indications of long-term benefit, Hydergine would seem to be of minor value in dementia therapy."* The results of more

---

*J. R. Hughes, J. G. Williams, and R. D. Currier. "An Ergot Alkaloid Preparation (Hydergine) in the Treatment of Dementia: Critical Review of the Clinical Literature." *Journal of American Geriatrics* 24: 490–97, 1976.

recent research in the intervening years does not contradict this judgment.

The effects of Hydergine in healthy people, also recommended by smart drug advocates, has received much less objective testing. Comments made in discussing the results of one series of trials is enlightening concerning the efficacy of Hydergine and also why, despite contradictory results, this drug continues to be advertised as helpful for aging people. A long-term study of a large number of healthy people, middle-aged and older, was undertaken in 1976. Hydergine's effectiveness on medical and cognitive processes was studied in a double-blind placebo-controlled trial. After five years, comparison of the people receiving Hydergine with those receiving the placebo, with respect to ten objectively measured medical and cognitive variables, revealed no effect of Hydergine. Yet despite this finding, the authors concluded, based on the fact that fewer people in the Hydergine group withdrew from the study due to illness and a variety of other similar findings, that this was "an argument in favor of a prophylactic effect of ergoloid mesylates on pathological concomitants of aging."* Such a conclusion, in the absence of a demonstrable effect of Hydergine on any of the objectively measured medical or cognitive indices, is hardly a ringing endorsement.

Hydergine has a low risk profile, with the most common side effects being nausea, insomnia, headache, and gastric distress.

---

*"Effects of Long-Term Ergoloid Mesylates (Hydergine) Administration in Healthy Pensioners: 5-Year Results." *Current Medical Research Opinion* 10: 256–79, 1986.

Typical dosages
Daily doses range from 3 mg to 9 mg.

Contraindications
Use of Hydergine is contraindicated in persons with psychosis or schizophrenia.

The plain facts
The scientific evidence supporting the advertised beneficial effects of Hydergine for healthy people or for those in early stages of senility is exceedingly weak. At best, this drug may have modest positive influences. The risks of Hydergine use do appear to be, as advertised, minimal.

Benefits: ½
Risks: 1

IDEBENONE
Nonprescription; available through Internet sources

What is it?
Idebenone, also known as Avan or Tap, is closely related to coenzyme Q-10, a critical cofactor in cellular energy metabolism controlled by the mitochondria. Idebenone is an antioxidant, free radical scavenger, and appears to enhance cerebral metabolism.

Its reputation
Idebenone is promoted as an antiaging compound that protects cognitive powers, particularly memory, against decline as we grow older.

The drug's effect on the brain
Idebenone may enhance cerebral metabolism as well as have antioxidant and free radical scavenging properties. These effects of idebenone suggest that this compound might have neuroprotective functions (i.e., the ability to protect brain cells from damage in certain pathological states). This suggestion was confirmed in experiments showing that idebenone kept neurons alive in conditions of low oxygen and decreased blood flow, as well as in the presence of toxic levels of glutamate and amyloid beta-peptide.

How has it been tested? What are the risks, if any?
Idebenone has been tested in the laboratory where, like other compounds described in this chapter that either did or did not benefit people, this particular drug helped rats to learn how to avoid a punishing shock. Testing in people has been much more limited. Searching through the literature revealed three double-blind placebo-controlled trials, each with large numbers of patients in the early stages of Alzheimer's disease. In each study, idebenone improved cognitive functioning and in two it was claimed that progression of the disease was slowed. Unfortunately, there have been no studies either of people with other types of neurodegenerative disease (e.g., cerebrovascular insufficiency) or of healthy people.

The risks of significant medical problems with the use of this drug have not been described. The most common side effects were nausea, stomach pain, increased liver enzymes, anxiety, insomnia, and dizziness. Due to the very limited testing of this drug in people, it is not known if other side effects are likely to be encountered.

Typical dosages

Dosages ranging from 30–300 mg per day were used in the clinical trials with beneficial effects noted at all dose levels.

Contraindications

There are no known contraindications.

The plain facts

The pharmacological properties (free radical scavenger, antioxidant) of idebenone that enable it to act as a neuroprotector suggest that it has potential in the treatment of certain neurodegenerative conditions. Thus, the promising results in the trials with Alzheimer's disease, although still preliminary, are encouraging but not altogether surprising. Whether or not idebenone's effects on the brain would be of any use to a young healthy adult is doubtful since the pernicious effects of free radicals and oxidative stress would not be expected to be significant at this stage of life. On the other hand, some have hypothesized that oxidative damage and free radicals become increasingly important as we age. If this is the case, idebenone should be considered to be a promising drug that deserves more testing but, in the absence of such data, is still a question mark for consumers.

Benefits: 1
Risks: 1

INDERAL

Prescription drug; available from Internet suppliers

What is it?

Inderal (propranalol hydrochloride) is a prescription drug commonly used to prevent migraines and to treat high blood pressure that, according to some, also is capable of increasing cognitive abilities under certain circumstances.

Its reputation

Some people's ability to think is adversely affected by stress. Such people, who typically described themselves as "not good in an emergency," have difficulties remembering information and making decisions when under pressure. It has been suggested that Inderal, because it blocks some of the body's normal reactions to stress, improves cognitive functioning in people who are sensitive to stress. "So propranalol is an intelligence increasing drug when used in situations where fear prevents one from thinking normally."*

The drug's effect on the brain

To understand how Inderal works, it is first necessary to describe the activities of adrenaline, a hormone/transmitter whose actions are partially blocked by Inderal. Under conditions of stress, adrenaline is released from the adrenal glands into the bloodstream, where it circulates to many organs of the body and also passes into the brain. Under the same conditions, adrenaline is also released from the axon terminals of certain neurons. Adrenaline affects many organs in the body, though Inderal is prescribed chiefly to counteract adrenaline's effects on blood vessels and the heart. Adrenaline raises blood pressure and increases heart rate; Inderal blocks these effects of adrenaline and thereby prevents the occurrence of some of the bodily reactions that people experience as feelings of anxiety. For this reason, Inderal makes some people feel more

---

*W. Dean and J. Morganthaler in *Smart Drugs*. Health Freedom Publications, 1991, p. 136.

calm in stressful situations. It is thought that Inderal enhances cognitive abilities by blocking the body's reactions to adrenaline and having a calming effect, rather than by direct influences on the brain's memory systems.

How has it been tested? What are the risks, if any?
Inderal's effects on cognition in general and memory in particular have been tested in at least twelve studies of varying scientific rigor. The principal support for the idea that this drug would enhance cognitive performance in stressful situations was a study in which high school students who complained of "stress-induced cognitive dysfunction" performed significantly better on retaking the SATs following administration of Inderal than they had when previously taking the examination without medication. Unfortunately, this study is not at all persuasive, since it was not done blind, did not use a placebo for comparison, and had no control group. In contrast, a placebo-controlled study of memory functioning in anxiety-provoking situations and a second study, double-blind and placebo-controlled, of memory function in patients with panic disorder showed that although Inderal had calming effects, it also impaired memory functioning. A tally of the effects of Inderal in nine other studies showed that enhancement of memory functioning was found in one experiment, impairment in four studies, and no effect in four others.

The risk potential of Inderal, a potent antagonist of one of the body's most important transmitters, is high (see contraindications). In addition to the problems associated with its use in contraindicated conditions and in drug interactions (see below), some of the more common side effects of this drug include diarrhea, weakness, lowered blood pressure, sleep disturbances, dizziness or lightheadedness, swelling in lower extremities, nightmares, and erectile dysfunction. This is definitely not a drug that should be taken without close supervision by a physician.

Typical dosages

Those who recommend the use of Inderal as a cognitive enhancer suggest a dosage of 10–30 mg be taken preferably after a meal and 1.5 hours before the stressful event. However, we must stress that, in view of the lack of evidence that it improves memory functioning under any conditions and its contraindications, we do not recommend the use of Inderal for cognitive enhancement.

Contraindications

Inderal is contraindicated in persons with a variety of heart problems, bronchospastic diseases (asthma, emphysema, chronic bronchitis), diabetes, hypoglycemia, certain types of thyroid problems, and persons with impaired kidney or liver functioning. In addition, Inderal interacts, sometimes fatally, with a variety of drugs used to treat psychiatric disorders (especially depression), calcium channel blockers, haloperidol, chlorpromazine, nonsteroidal anti-inflammatory agents (e.g., ibuprofen) and Tagamet. If you are contemplating taking Inderal, a physician should be consulted to determine if there are additional contraindications or drug interactions that should be considered in your specific case.

The plain facts

Although Inderal is a potent drug that has many effects on the body, there is no convincing evidence that cognitive enhancement, in stressful or other conditions, is included among its actions. In view of Inderal's side effects, contraindications, and drug interactions, the risk/benefit ratio is not stacked in favor of taking this drug for its rumored positive influences on memory.

Benefits: ½
Risks: 5

NIMODIPINE
Prescription drug; available through Internet suppliers

What is it?
Nimodipine, also known as Nimotop, belongs to the class of drugs known as calcium channel blockers. Calcium serves many crucial biological functions in the body. Nimodipine, a prescription drug in the United States, was designed with the intent of affecting calcium's actions in the muscles that line the blood vessels. In this smooth muscle, calcium enters the fibers of the muscle through microscopic pores, called calcium channels, and thereby allows these muscles to contract. Nimodipine, by blocking these channels, prevents excessive contractions of blood vessels. This drug is intended for treatment of patients who have suffered ruptured blood vessels in the brain where it is hoped that nimodipine will prevent spasms of other blood vessels. It has also been found to be useful in useful in reducing cluster and migraine headaches. Its uses in cognitive enhancement were discovered only secondarily.

Its reputation
Nimodipine is thought to enhance memory due to an ability to keep the brain's blood vessels dilated and thereby increase

blood flow to the brain. In addition, it has been suggested that this drug also increases the production of acetylcholine, a neurotransmitter some consider to be especially important for memory formation.

The drug's effect on the brain
There is no evidence that nimodipine increases blood flow to the brain in healthy people nor is there evidence that this drug increases acetylcholine levels. Indeed, in some brain areas nimodipine actually decreases the release of acetyl-choline. In any case, it would be highly unlikely that effects on cerebral circulation or selective enhancement acetyl-choline production would be of much use to healthy people. Maintaining optimal blood flow to the brain is biologically the highest priority; when pressed in an emergency, the body will sacrifice all of the organs but the heart in an effort to keep the brain adequately supplied with blood. Acetylcholine is probably involved in memory formation but not more so than other neurotransmitters such as glutamate, gamma-aminobutyric acid (GABA), dopamine, and probably dozens if not hundreds more. Even if acetylcholine was a special and singular "memory" transmitter, just the semblance of a rea-sonable diet in a healthy person is sufficient to keep the brain supplied with adequate levels of acetylcholine. Thus, if nimodipine has beneficial effects on cognition, some other(s) of its actions must be the basis.

It is most likely that nimodipine's ability to block calcium channels underlies its positive effects. Disruption of calcium homeostasis in the brain is a common accompaniment of aging. In addition, increased flow of calcium into brain cells contributes to a pathological process called excitotoxicity, one of the primary mechanisms underlying the death of neurons in head trauma, stroke, many neurodegenerative diseases, and, possibly, during aging.

How has it been tested? What are the risks, if any?
Nimodipine has been tested in laboratory research and been shown to have a variety of positive effects that may be relevant to people. This drug lessened the severity of neurological impairments following experimentally induced stroke in rats. In addition, nimodipine improved learning and memory in aging rats and rabbits. But does nimodipine have positive effects in people?

The effects of nimodipine have been tested in three patient groups; those with cardiac problems, stroke patients, and people in early stages of dementia. Due to transient loss of oxygen to the brain, many persons (50 percent) who have suffered cardiac arrest and then been resuscitated will experience moderate to severe cognitive problems for at least a year. Single dose injection of nimodipine following cardiac arrest did not improve cognitive outcome. In another study, patients undergoing heart surgery requiring cardiopulmonary bypass were studied in a double-blind placebo-controlled experiment. Persisting memory problems are a frequent complaint following cardiopulmonary bypass. Patients who had received nimodipine performed better on tests of verbal fluency and also visual memory. These positive effects of nimodipine cannot be attributed to effects on circulation since there were no differences in measures of cerebral blood flow between the groups that received the drug and those that were administered placebo.

For the same reasons that cardiac patients have cognitive problems (i.e., oxygen deprivation), patients who have suffered a stroke are subject to many of the same difficulties. It was shown in a single-blind placebo-controlled study that patients receiving nimodipine daily for three months following their stroke have better memory functioning than those who received placebo.

The effects of nimodipine on cognitive functioning in patients with dementia were tested in three open and two double-blind placebo-controlled trials. Each of these studies had similar results: nimodipine improved memory, attention, and overall cognitive functioning.

The main risk associated with use of nimodipine is decreased blood pressure; clearly this drug should not be used in conjunction with other calcium blockers (e.g., verapamil), beta blockers, or antihypertensives. Other adverse reactions include slowing of heart rate, headache, nausea, depression, muscle pain, skin rash, and acne. Since this is a prescription drug, a comprehensive list of nimodipine's potential side effects can be found in the *Physicians' Desk Reference*, available in most reference libraries. However, due to nimodipine's potential to influence many functions important to sustain life, a physician should be consulted before initiating treatment.

Typical dosages
Ninety mg administered daily in three divided doses was used in the majority of clinical trials described here. In *Smart Drugs*, the authors advise: "For cognition enhancement purposes in otherwise healthy individuals it may be best to start with a small fraction of the normal 30 mg capsule or tablet."

Contraindications
There are no known contraindications.

The plain facts

Nimodipine is a calcium channel blocker that has been shown to protect cognitive functions in various pathological states. On the other hand, there are no studies that suggest cognitive enhancing effects of this drug in healthy people. Indeed, if its positive effects on cognition in cardiac, stroke, and dementia patients are due to protection against excitotoxicity, nimodipine would not improve memory in healthy people; excitotoxicity is a pathological process common to injury and disease. In view of nimodipine's powerful effects on the cardiovascular and other organ systems, use of this drug for cognitive enhancement in healthy people, particularly if unsupervised by a physician, is ill advised.

Benefits: 2
Risks: 4

ONDANSETRON
Prescription drug; not found on Internet yet

What is it?

Ondansetron, marketed as the prescription drug Zofran, is an antiemetic, a drug used to combat nausea. It works by blocking some of the actions of the neurotransmitter serotonin.

Its reputation

Ondansetron is thought to have memory enhancing effects in addition to its well-documented antiemetic efficacy. This drug is also thought to be useful for reducing feelings of anxiety.

The drug's effect on the brain

Ondansetron is reputed to improve memory through indirect actions on the neurotransmitter acetylcholine. Some neurons that release serotonin from their axon terminals suppress the activity of other brain cells that release acetylcholine. Blockade of serotonin's suppressive action, by administration of ondansetron, allows the brain cells containing acetylcholine to release more of their transmitter. Since some hypothesize that acetylcholine has a special role in memory, they speculate that facilitation of acetylcholine release will facilitate the formation of memory. Findings from research using laboratory animals are supportive of these ideas since ondansetron can reverse the negative effects of acetylcholine blockade on learning and also exerts facilitatory influences on some types of learning and memory in normal animals.

How has it been tested? What are the risks, if any?

Ondansetron has not been tested in patients with Alzheimer's disease or with other forms of dementia. However, there have been several double-blind placebo-controlled trials of this drug's effects in normal young adults and healthy elderly people. Neither positive nor negative effects were found; ondansetron appeared to have no effects on cognitive processes including memory.

Side effects of ondansetron include headache, general malaise, fatigue, weakness, gastrointestinal problems (stomach pain, constipation, or diarrhea), and dizziness.

Typical dosages

When used to combat nausea, 8 mg ondansetron tablets are taken three times a day. No dosage recommendations for use in cognitive enhancement are reported since no data supports such a use.

Contraindications

Ondansetron should not be used by individuals who have had allergic reactions to related drugs (such as granisetron or dolasetron) or who are pregnant or breast-feeding. In addition, patients with liver disease may have an increased chance of side effects.

The plain facts

There is no solid evidence that ondansetron has beneficial effects on memory or aspects of cognition. Based on currently available information, there is no rationale for using this drug for its effects on cognition.

Benefits: 0
Risks: 2

OXIRACETAM
Nonprescription drug; available through Internet suppliers

What is it?

Oxiracetam (also known as Neuroactiv and Neuromet) is one of the nootropics, drugs designed solely for cognitive enhancing effects. This particular drug is one of a family of racetams (i.e., pramiracetam, etiracetam, aniracetam, rolziracetam), drugs that resemble piracetam, the first of the nootropics (discussed elsewhere in this chapter).

Its reputation

Oxiracetam is advertised as a drug that enhances memory abilities in normal people and in patients in the early stages of senile dementia. Although not yet approved by the FDA for use in the United States, it is widely used in Europe. In addition, this drug is reputed to be devoid of serious side effects or contraindications.

The drug's effect on the brain

It is not known how oxiracetam or any of the other drugs in the racetam family work or what their effects are in the brain. Although for some of the racetams (e.g., piracetam), theories have been advanced, there has been little hypothesized concerning oxiracetam.

How has it been tested? What are the risks, if any?

Oxiracetam has been tested extensively in groups of patients with memory problems due to degenerative disease. It has been shown to improve memory and attention in seven of eight double-blind placebo-controlled trials on groups of patients with Alzheimer's disease, multi-infarct dementia, and dementia of unspecified origin. Positive effects were seen with daily administrations lasting a month to one year.

Unfortunately, there have been no double-blind placebo-controlled studies in healthy individuals, whether young, middle-aged, or elderly. Since, as discussed in Chapter 2, the causes of memory and other cognitive problems in patients with degenerative diseases such as Alzheimer's can be quite different from those in healthy people, treatments that are effective in disease-related cognitive problems will not necessarily be efficacious in healthy persons.

Oxiracetam's reputed safety has been borne out in many studies in which side effects, none serious, are reported by only a few of the people receiving the drug. This low incidence of side effects and adverse reactions was maintained with chronic daily dosage lasting as long as one year.

Typical dosages
Commercial suppliers suggest a dosage range of 1,200–2,400 mg daily. In many of the clinical trials in which oxiracetam was shown to be effective in Alzheimer's and other demented patients, 1,600 mg per day, in two divided doses, was used.

Contraindications
There are no known contraindications for the use of oxiracetam.

The plain facts
Oxiracetam's reputed effectiveness as a safe memory enhancer in Alzheimer's patients is well supported by sound clinical trials. In contrast, there is no evidence yet concerning its beneficial effects in normal people. This drug is used extensively in Italy but has not yet been approved for use in the United States. FDA approval is being sought by a major drug company for use of oxiracetam with Alzheimer's patients.

Benefits: 2½
Risks: ½

PHOSPHATIDYLSERINE

(Dietary supplement; available over the counter in specialty stores, pharmacies, supermarkets, and through Internet suppliers)

What is it?
Neurons are cells that, like all of the cells in the body, are surrounded by a cell membrane composed of lipids (fats)

and proteins. Phosphatidylserine, a lipid, is rapidly incorporated into the cell membranes of neurons where it affects certain types of neurotransmitter receptors (see Chapter 3, Figure 3).

Its reputation

Phosphatidylserine is advertised as a cognitive enhancer that works by augmenting the brain's metabolic rate and also by facilitating synaptic communication between brain cells. Commercial suppliers suggest that the brain's phosphatidylserine levels decrease as we age and, as a result, memory suffers.

The drug's effect on the brain

A variety of studies showed that phosphatidylserine facilitated mice in learning to avoid an electric shock and, in addition, counteracted the deleterious influences of lowering rats' acetylcholine levels on their ability to remember what they had recently learned. One interpretation of these findings was that phosphatidylserine's positive effects were based upon an ability to raise the brain's acetylcholine levels. If this is the case phosphatidylserine would be of little benefit for healthy people since acetylcholine levels would not be abnormally low in the absence of illness. However, phosphatidylserine also increases the activity of specific types of receptors that are sensitive to glutamate, a neurotransmitter that is involved in many behavioral functions including learning and memory. In addition, this lipid increases the brain's metabolic rate and facilitates synaptic transmission involving the neurotransmitter dopamine.

Phosphatidylserine may also have indirect effects on the brain through influences on hormonal systems. As discussed in Chapter 3, stress and the principal hormone secreted during stress, cortisol, have negative influence on cognitive abilities in general and memory in particular. Phosphatidylserine dampens the body's response to stress and decreases the secretion of cortisol.

How has it been tested? What are the risks, if any?
The results of studies investigating phosphatidylserine's influences on cognition have been remarkably consistent. In several double-blind placebo-controlled trials using either senile patients or healthy elderly people experiencing mild memory problems, phosphatidylserine improved neuropsychological functioning including memory and attention. In addition to these positive results, adverse reactions to phosphatidylserine were exceedingly rare.

Typical dosages
Three hundred mg/day, in three divided doses, was administered orally in the trials in which cognitive functioning was improved.

Contraindications
There are some indications that phosphatidylserine slows blood coagulation. For this reason it may be contraindicated for persons with clotting disorders, such as hemophilia, as well as persons taking anticoagulants, such as Coumadin or aspirin therapy.

The plain facts
If you do not have a contraindicated condition, phosphatidylserine is a relatively safe substance that has positive effects on attention and memory in both healthy individuals and those in the early stages of senility.

Benefits: 4
Risks: ½

PIRACETAM
Nonprescription drug; available through Internet suppliers

What is it?
Piracetam is part of the family of racetams, and is similar in molecular structure to the amino acid pyroglutamate. Piracetam, also known as Nootropil, was the first nootropic drug to be marketed in Europe.

Its reputation
Piracetam is advertised as a way to "boost intelligence," to improve memory, learning, and possibly, to enhance creativity. In addition, piracetam is suggested to have these beneficial effects without either toxic side effects or addictive potential. Although the ways in which piracetam is purported to accomplish these effects is not known, there is no shortage of theories. For example, it has been advertised that piracetam stimulates the cerebral cortex and increases the rate of metabolism and energy level of neurons. In addition, it has been said that this drug also facilitates the flow of information between the right and left hemispheres of the brain and also improves the functioning of the neurotransmitter acetylcholine.

The drug's effect on the brain
In actual fact, the real scientific evidence supporting each of the theories mentioned above of how piracetam works is, at best, exceedingly weak and, more typically, virtually nonex-

istent. However, is it really important to understand the biological effects of a drug if the use of that drug has beneficial effects and there are no adverse side effects? The history of medicine is full of examples in which drugs are accepted by the medical community and widely used despite ignorance of how their positive effects are achieved. It is only in the past decade that we have gained a basic understanding of aspirin's painkilling ability and its amazing anti-inflammatory effects, although it has been widely used since the turn of the twentieth century. Major tranquilizers, the only drugs that help alleviate the symptoms of schizophrenia, have been widely prescribed since the mid-1950s yet the basis of their beneficial effects remains a matter of dispute even today.

How has it been tested? What are the risks, if any?
There are a multitude of studies in which piracetam improves brain functioning and facilitates learning and memory in mice and rats. Many of these studies are well designed and published in respected scientific journals. However, for reasons that were described in Chapter 1, the best way to evaluate a drug's effect on thinking ability is with double-blind placebo-controlled studies in people. In such a study of persons in an early stage of Alzheimer's disease, published in a reputable neurological journal, piracetam appeared to slightly slow the rate at which patients' short-term and long-term memory deteriorated. However, memory loss in Alzheimer's disease is due to the progressive death of neurons. Memory problems in neurologically normal people probably do not result from the same process as in patients with Alzheimer's or other forms of senility. It is therefore more significant that two double-blind placebo-

controlled studies of patients with what was described as "age associated memory impairment" showed significant improvement in memory if given piracetam in combination with memory training. Either piracetam or memory training in isolation was also beneficial, albeit less so than the combined treatment.

Piracetam has also been tested on children with dyslexia. Although there is not total agreement, the majority of double-blind placebo-controlled studies, and there have been quite a few, showed improvement in reading performance while on the drug.

Typical dosages

Piracetam is available as either capsules or tablets in doses of 400 and 800 mg. The typical dose range is a total of 2,400 to 4,800 mg per day taken in three divided doses.

Contraindications

There are no known contraindications to the use of piracetam.

The plain facts

Reports of any untoward effects of piracetam are extremely rare. Considering the extensive testing of piracetam in normal and neurologically impaired adults as well as in dyslexic children, this is an impressive and reassuring consistency. In summary, there is some indication that piracetam improves memory. In addition, there have been no reports to date that this drug carries a risk of any serious side effect.

Benefits: 2½
Risks: ½

PRAMIRACETAM
Nonprescription drug; available through Internet suppliers

What is it?
Pramiracetam is one of the family of racetams, made up of structurally similar compounds such as etiracetam, aniracetam, and rolziracetam, drugs that resemble piracetam, the first of the nootropics.

Its reputation
Pramiracetam is reputed to be a memory enhancing agent that is similar in actions to piracetam but is more powerful.

The drug's effect on the brain
The effects of this drug on the brain, like the other racetam nootropics, are still not known. Some influences on the acetylcholine in various parts of the brain, including the cortex and hippocampus, have been reported in studies on rats. Pramiracetam has been shown to be without effect on other transmitter systems, including GABA, dopamine, norepinephrine, and serotonin.

How has it been tested? What are the risks, if any?
There has been only very limited testing in people. Although positive effects on memory functioning in Alzheimer's patients was found in an open trial, an attempt to confirm this beneficial effect in a double-blind placebo-controlled trial was unsuccessful. While no assessment of this drug's effects on healthy people, either young or elderly, has been published, there was a double-blind placebo-controlled trial using young men suffering memory problems as a result of head injury. Pramiracetam

had clear beneficial effects on the recovery of memory functioning in these brain injured patients.

Pramiracetam, like its close cousin piracetam, appears to be quite safe. Significant side effects were not reported in the clinical trials.

Typical dosages

Doses used in the clinical trials varied from 400 to 4,000 mg per day. In the study of memory recovery after head injury, 400 mg tablets were taken three times each day.

Contraindications

There are no known contraindications.

The plain facts

Pramiracetam appears to be similar to piracetam at least in respect to its lack of significant side effects. Unlike piracetam, however, it has not been well studied and its only clear beneficial effects on memory were seen in head injured patients. Until more data concerning the efficacy of this drug becomes available, there is not sufficient objective information to justify its use in either healthy people or those with early senility.

Benefits: 1½
Risks: 1

VINCAMINE

Herbal dietary supplement; available over the counter or through Internet suppliers

---

What is it?

Vincamine is an alkaloid derived from the periwinkle plant and is thought to increase blood flow to the brain. It is sold in Europe under a variety of names.

Its reputation

Vincamine is advertised as a safe drug that, in healthy people, will improve the ability to concentrate and, in persons with cognitive problems due to impaired circulation to/in the brain (cerebrovascular insufficiency), will enhance memory and attention.

The drug's effect on the brain

In experiments in laboratory animals and also in clinical trials using stroke patients, this drug clearly increases blood flow to the brain. If given soon after the occurrence of a stroke, the patient's movement problems and difficulties with sphincter control show increased recovery. The effects of vincamine are not confined to blood flow, however. This drug blocks the flow of the ion sodium into cells, an action that could protect brain cells in certain pathological states but would decrease excitability under normal conditions. Vincamine also increases the activity of brain cells that release norepinephrine in an area of the brain stem called the locus coeruleus. Increased activity in the locus coeruleus may enhance attention but has negative implications for normal sleep patterns. Locus coeruleus must cease activity in order for the REM stage of sleep to occur.

How has it been tested? What are the risks, if any?

Vincamine helps rats to learn how to avoid punishment and counteracts the disruptive effects on learning of either decreasing the brain's acetylcholine activity or of drug-induced seizures. There have been several clinical trials in which patients suffering cognitive problems due to cerebrovascular insufficiency were administered vincamine with generally positive results. In two open and in four double-blind placebo-controlled trials, statistically significant improvements were seen in memory and attentional functioning. The potential benefits of vincamine for other groups of people are unknown; there have been no reports of trials using Alzheimer's patients or healthy people.

Although vincamine is promoted as a safe drug, it is not. With short-term use there have been few reports of adverse effects but with repeated administrations the picture is more disturbing. Significant disruptions of the heart's activity (severe cardiac arrhythmia) has been attributed to vincamine, an adverse effect that can be lethal. While several predisposing factors have been suggested (see Contraindications following), these arrhythmias have also been seen in people assumed to have been healthy. Vincamine also disrupts sleep patterns, particularly the REM stage, an action that is predictable based on this drug's effects on norepinephrine.

Typical dosages
Dosages range up to a maximum of 120 mg per day.

Contraindications
The use of vincamine is contraindicated for persons with atrial fibrillation, ventricular tachycardia or any other cardiac arrhythmia, cardiomegaly, or chronic obstructive airway disease, and people suffering from sleep disturbances.

The plain facts

Vincamine appears to be useful for patients suffering cognitive problems due to cerebrovascular insufficiency. There is no evidence of effectiveness for either Alzheimer's patients or for healthy people with mild cognitive difficulties. It is also stressed that vincamine is not a safe drug and should not be used unless under the direct supervision of an appropriately trained health professional.

Benefits: 0

Risks: 5

VINPOCETINE

Herbal dietary supplement; available over the counter or through Internet suppliers

---

What is it?

Vinpocetine, also known as Cavinton, is derived from vincamine (see preceding), a product of the periwinkle plant. Vinpocetine acts as a vasodilator, though it also has other effects, and has been used in Europe to treat victims of stroke.

Its reputation

Vinpocetine is heralded not only as a safe and reliable treatment for problems due to poor circulation to the brain, but also as an aid for the memory problems of healthy individuals. Promotional literature states that the beneficial effects of this drug are supported by the published results of over a hundred clinical trials.

The drug's effect on the brain

Vinpocetine's ability to increase blood flow to the brain has been well documented in experiments involving laboratory animals and also in clinical trials with people. Effects on cerebral blood flow are not, however, the only influences of this drug on the brain. Vinpocetine, in certain pathological conditions, blocks the flow of sodium and calcium into brain cells and thereby prevents damage and acts as a "neuroprotectant." It has been suggested that this effect, rather than its influence on cerebral blood flow, is the basis of its beneficial influences on the brain.

How has it been tested? What are the risks, if any?

There have been a sufficient number of well-designed studies of vinpocetine's effects on rats to establish that the drug enhanced learning to avoid punishment and counteracted the amnesia-producing influences of experimentally lowering acetylcholine in the brain. The situation concerning the evaluation of its effectiveness in people is quite different, however.

Despite the advertising copy suggesting that there are numerous published studies of vinpocetine's effectiveness in people, the reality appears to be quite different. The situation is aptly summarized in a recent review of trials testing vinpocetine's effectiveness in preventing death following stroke. The authors searched through MEDLINE's 9.2 million plus articles from international biomedical journals, and contacted the manufacturers of vinpocetine for all available information concerning trials. To be included in the review, the study had to use objective measures in a double-blind placebo-controlled trial. "Among the identified studies on vinpocetine in stroke, only one fulfilled the selection criteria."[*]

---

[*]D. Bereczki and I. Fekete. "A Systematic Review of Vinpocetine Therapy in Acute Ischemic Stroke." *European Journal of Pharmacology* 55: 349–52, 1999.

In examining the medical literature concerning the cognitive enhancing effects of vinpocetine, we met with similarly disappointing results. Only two double-blind placebo-controlled trials tested this drug's effects in senile patients. Both showed improved cognitive functioning but only one of these trials specifically tested memory abilities. There was only one double-blind placebo-controlled test of vinpocetine's effects in healthy people. This trial, although reporting improved short-term memory, tested too few people (twelve) to allow any conclusions to be drawn.

The incidence of adverse reactions with the use of vinpocetine is low. A negative influence on blood clotting seems to be present although it is reported to be mild.

Typical dosages
Dosages from 5–60 mg per day have been reported. In clinical trials, daily doses of either 30 mg or 60 mg, each in three divided doses, were often used.

Contraindications
Persons with clotting disorders and patients taking Coumadin or aspirin therapy should consult their doctor before taking vinpocetine.

The plain facts
Vinpocetine is a heavily promoted drug that seems to be safe but has only sparse objective evidence to support the expansive claims made concerning its beneficial effects on memory in senile and healthy people. Its documented biological actions as a neuroprotective agent and also its ability to increase blood flow to the brain suggest that this drug might be potentially helpful to persons with certain types of brain

disorders. On the other hand, whether vinpocetine's known actions would be of any help to healthy people can only be conjectured in the absence of scientific evidence.

Benefits: ½
Risks: 1½

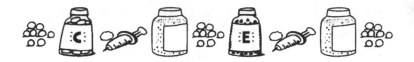

5

Amino Acids

Amino acids are a diverse class of carbon-containing (organic) molecules that serve many biological functions that are crucial to basic operations of the body. Although it is generally known that amino acids are the building blocks of proteins, certain of these important molecules also act as neurotransmitters in the brain. For example, the amino acid glutamate is the most common neurotransmitter in the brain by which one neuron can excite its neighbor. Another amino acid called gamma-aminobutyric acid, or GABA for short, is the most common transmitter in the brain that can dampen (inhibit) the actions of adjacent neurons. In view of the fundamental importance of these compounds to brain functioning, it is not surprising that drugs targeted at amino acids are thought to have effects on one of the primary activities of the brain: cognition. This chapter will review the evidence suggesting that these drugs actually work and will discuss the possible risks.

ACETYL-L-CARNITINE

Dietary supplement; available over the counter and through Internet suppliers

What is it?

To understand what acetyl-l-carnitine is, it is first necessary to describe the functions of mitochondria. Mitochondria are organelles, that is, differentiated structures within a living cell that perform a specific function. The function of mitochondria is to provide the energy that fuels virtually all of the cell's activities. In brain cells, energy metabolism by mitochondria allows neurons to, among other things, produce neurotransmitters, support the electrical activity that is the basis for communication, repair themselves when damaged, and store information. Typically, as some people age, energy production by mitochondria becomes less efficient. Some researchers think that with declining mitochondrial functioning comes an increased susceptibility of neurons to damage by free radicals and an erosion of cognitive abilities. In normal functioning, the amino acid L-carnitine, both derived from food and also synthesized in the liver and kidneys, enables the mitochondria to use fatty acids for energy production. It is thought that acetyl-l-carnitine, closely related to L-carnitine, performs the same function.

Its reputation

Acetyl-l-carnitine is promoted as a supplement based on its advertised ability to energize the brain, improve memory and attention in young healthy people, and to fight off the effects of aging. In addition, retailers tout its beneficial effects in Alzheimer's disease, depression, alcohol-induced cognitive impairments, and Down's syndrome.

The drug's effect on the brain

Laboratory research has shown that acetyl-l-carnitine does indeed have a number of effects in the brain that are of potential benefit to people. As advertised, acetyl-l-carnitine does increase energy metabolism in brain cells. In addition, this amino acid appears to have neuroprotective activity during several types of pathological conditions. For example, it promotes brain cell survival during the period of oxygen deprivation caused by interruption of blood circulation to the brain and also during the oxidative stress that occurs when circulation is restored. Acetyl-l-carnitine also helps brain cells to recover from physical damage. Ordinarily, a high proportion of neurons will die after experimental axotomy (cutting off the neuron's axon). In the presence of acetyl-l-carnitine, a higher percentage of axotomized neurons recover and regenerate new axons. This amino acid also protected the developing learning abilities of mice that had been exposed to alcohol in utero. Finally, of possible direct relevance to Alzheimer's patients, acetyl-l-carnitine helps brain cells to overcome the toxic effects of exposure to beta amyloid. Beta amyloid is a protein that is the primary constituent of neuritic plaques, one of the two types of brain lesions that proliferate in the brains of Alzheimer's patients.

How has it been tested? What are the risks, if any?

The effects of acetyl-l-carnitine on patients with mental decline due to Alzheimer's disease, cerebrovascular insufficiency, and other age-related forms of neural deterioration have been extensively tested in double-blind placebo-controlled studies. Beneficial effects of this amino acid on memory, attention, verbal fluency, and executive functioning have been consistently reported, with trials of supplementation lasting as few as thirty days and as long as one year. There was some evidence that the benefit was greatest in either younger Alzheimer's patients or those with earlier disease onset.

One double-blind placebo-controlled trial evaluated acetyl-l-carnitine's supposed positive effects on the cognitive impairments caused by chronic alcoholism. In this large study, ninety days of drug treatment was sufficient to improve memory and executive functioning in abstinent alcoholics.

It has also been suggested that acetyl-l-carnitine is beneficial to cognitive functioning in adults with Down's syndrome. Since adults with Down's syndrome develop Alzheimer's pathology in their brains and, as discussed, this amino acid is beneficial to Alzheimer's patients, it is plausible that this drug will also be effective in Down's patients. A search through the literature failed to turn up sufficiently objective trials to evaluate acetyl-l-carnitine's efficacy with Down's patients. However, what little evidence that is available (i.e., an open study) does suggest that acetyl-l-carnitine has potential benefit.

There are also claims that acetyl-l-carnitine improves mood in depressed patients. Although there were several studies that supported such an effect in nondemented patients, these trials were either not placebo controlled or clearly double-blind. As a result, the beneficial influences on depression remains to be objectively evaluated.

Acetyl-l-carnitine appears to be quite safe; review of seventeen clinical trials failed to reveal side effects more significant than nausea or a few isolated cases of vomiting. A cautionary note is in order, however. The related compound, DL-carnitine, is sold over the counter in some health food stores and can produce a loss of muscular strength similar to that of myasthenia gravis. This pathological condition results because DL-carnitine interferes with the functions of L-carnitine in the mitochondria.

Typical dosages
Doses as high as 3 grams per day were used in some clinical trials, though beneficial effects were typically seen with 1 to 1.5 grams daily.

Contraindications
There are no contraindications for the use of acetyl-l-carnitine.

The plain facts
Acetyl-l-carnitine is a safe and effective drug to treat the cognitive impairments associated with Alzheimer's disease and other age-related forms of cognitive deterioration. Based on this amino acid's pharmacological actions, it is at least plausible that it would also be beneficial for the more benign memory problems associated with aging in healthy people. On the other hand, there is neither evidence nor a rationale for the use of acetyl-l-carnitine in young healthy individuals.

Benefits: 2½
Risks: ½

MILACEMIDE
Nonprescription drug; available through Internet suppliers

What is it?
While Milacemide is not an amino acid, it acts similarly to glycine in the brain. Glycine is an amino acid that functions

as a neurotransmitter at two types of receptors in synapses. First, there are specialized glycine receptors in the spinal cord whose functions are not understood at this time. Secondly, glycine has an important influence on NMDA receptors. These receptors must be affected by both glutamate and glycine acting in concert in order for activation to occur. NMDA receptors are thought to be involved in many behavioral processes including memory and learning.

Its reputation

It is advertised that this drug improves memory and attention in both normal people and in Alzheimer's disease patients.

The drug's effect on the brain

Because of the way this drug affects the brain, claims have been made that it can improve cognitive functioning. Milacemide's actions are thought to follow from its ability to increase the brain's levels of the amino acid neurotransmitter, glycine. As a prerequisite to understanding glycine's actions, one must first know a little more about neurotransmitters and receptors.

Once a neurotransmitter is released into the synapse (discussed in more detail in Chapter 3), it floats across the space between neurons (synaptic cleft) until it contacts a specialized area of the adjacent neuron, the receptor, that is sensitive to that particular transmitter. One type of receptor that is responsive to glycine is called the NMDA receptor. Activation of NMDA receptors may be particularly relevant to the actions of smart drugs because these types of receptors seem to "learn" from past experience. Once a neuron with NMDA receptors is activated by other neurons showing a particular pattern of firing, it remains more easily excited by those neurons for an extended period of time. Scientists who study how the brain stores memories believe that similar types of changes in neuron activity caused by NMDA receptors are an important part of the process that allows the brain to store information.

The rationale behind the use of Milacemide is that increasing glycine levels will augment NMDA activity and thereby facilitate the formation of memory. Glycine itself cannot be given because, once absorbed into the blood, it is blocked from entering the brain by the blood-brain barrier. In contrast, Milacemide readily crosses the blood-brain barrier, where it is quickly converted by the brain into glycine. Does this have any effect on memory?

How has it been tested? What are the risks, if any?
Milacemide, like many drugs thought to have cognitive enhancing properties, has been well tested on patients with memory impairment associated with Alzheimer's disease. Three well-designed double-blind placebo-controlled investigations, performed by different groups of scientists and published in first-rank medical journals, demonstrated that Milacemide had no effect on any measure of cognitive functioning in these individuals. These results are particularly convincing because very large numbers of patients were evaluated. It should be noted, however, that lack of efficacy in Alzheimer's patients does not necessarily rule out the possibility of a beneficial cognitive effect in healthy individuals. Memory problems in Alzheimer's disease are caused by the death of neurons in the parts of the brain that store information; a similar process is not responsible for the milder memory problems that most healthy people experience as they get older.

At least four investigations of Milacemide's effects in

healthy people suggested beneficial effects on some aspect of cognition. One of the earliest studies of Milacemide's cognitive effects in normal individuals showed improvements of attention and concentration. Although double-blind and placebo-controlled, the number of people evaluated was small (twelve) and the results appeared in a second-tier medical journal. A subsequent investigation, performed by the same scientists, evaluated Milacemide's effects using "elderly" (late sixties), and presumably healthy, people. In this trial, like the first, only twelve people were tested and the design was double-blind and placebo-controlled. However, stronger positive effects were found in these older subjects, with improvement observed in memory and attention and also in feelings of general well-being. Two additional double-blind placebo-controlled investigations were performed in groups of healthy young and older subjects and, again, increases of memory performance were observed.

Unfortunately, the pronouncement by some smart drug advocates that Milacemide appears to have minimal toxicity is seriously inaccurate. Experimental work using laboratory animals suggested the possibility that this drug could damage the liver. These fears were borne out in two clinical trials in which Milacemide was used for one month in Alzheimer's disease patients. With this short-term chronic use, Milacemide resulted in abnormalities in liver function in about 4 percent of subjects in each study. These liver abnormalities were deemed significant enough to cause termination of drug treatment.

In addition to liver problems, Milacemide may also have neurological risks. Milacemide worsens the abnormal movements that are the symptoms of Parkinson's disease. In addition, because Milacemide probably activates NMDA receptors, there are other dangers that may far outweigh possible toxic effects on the liver. Under normal conditions, NMDA receptors are the source of excitatory communication between countless neurons in the brain. However, under certain conditions, overstimulation of NMDA receptors leads to a pathological state wherein neurons are killed by a process called excitotoxicity. Since Milacemide increases glycine levels in the brain, which in turn leads to NMDA stimulation, a very real possibility exists, particularly with long-term treatment and high dose levels, of overstimulating NMDA receptors and inducing excitotoxicity.

Typical dosages
In the majority of the scientific studies of Milacemide, the daily dose range was 400–1,200 mg daily, although a few trials used doses as high as 1,600 mg.

Contraindications
Milacemide is contraindicated for persons with liver disease (e.g., cirrhosis, hepatitis) and Parkinson's disease patients. In addition, persons with other disorders of the basal ganglia such as Tourette's syndrome should discuss the use of Milacemide with their neurologist before attempting its use.

The plain facts
Milacemide appears to enhance attention and/or memory in healthy individuals while having no beneficial effect in ameliorating the cognitive symptoms of Alzheimer's disease patients. The positive influences of this drug should be weighed against its potential for adversely affecting liver function and its as yet undetermined risk of neurological toxicity.

Benefits: 2
Risks: 4

PYROGLUTAMATE
Dietary supplement; available over the counter and through Internet suppliers

What is it?
Pyroglutamate is an amino acid found in a variety of foods including dairy products, meat, fruit, and vegetables.

Its reputation
Pyroglutamate is reputed to enhance cognitive functioning in healthy people with age-related memory problems as well as sufferers from various forms of senility (e.g., Alzheimer's disease, multi-infarct dementia) and alcoholism.

The drug's effect in the brain
It is unclear how pyroglutamate got its reputation as a cognitive enhancer or what is the rationale for its use. The retailers of pyroglutamate offer neither explanations nor theories. The absence of even speculation is an unusual occurrence in the smart drug business since ordinarily, in the absence of solid or even not-so-solid information, at least some manufacturers will over-interpret a study of drug effects in mice or rats to generate a fanciful basis for advertising wonderful benefits to people. The fact that the basis of pyroglutamate's supposed benefits is not part of the advertisements indicates the singular paucity of information concerning the actions of this amino acid in the brain.

There is limited information on pyroglutamate's effects on brain chemistry. This amino acid is structurally related to glutamate, an excitatory neurotransmitter found in high concentrations throughout the brain. Several studies have shown that pyroglutamate can affect glutamate receptors and possibly block the actions of glutamate at these sites.

Other work has indicated that pyroglutamate can increase the brain's metabolism and cerebral blood flow. Unfortunately, these effects are not necessarily either beneficial or detrimental. Any drug that increases the activity of brain cells will increase their need for fuel and thereby increase the brain's metabolism and cerebral blood flow. Even toxic agents, if they are stimulants, would have this effect. Thus, rat poison containing strychnine, because it increases brain cell activity, could be expected to increase the brain's metabolism and cerebral blood flow!

How has it been tested? What are the risks, if any?

There are several studies of pyroglutamate's effects on learning and memory in laboratory rats. This drug facilitates learning in aged rats and counteracts the disruptive effects of other drugs that interfere with acetylcholine's effects in the brain. It should be noted that these experiments studied short-term administration of pyroglutamate.

Review of the scientific and medical literature disclosed only one double-blind placebo-controlled trial of pyroglutamate's effects in people. In this very small study, in which only twenty people received the drug, improvements in verbal memory in people suffering from age-related memory decline were reported.

Because of the lack of clinical trials, the risks of pyroglutamate are presently uncharted. However, if pyroglutamate is, in fact, an effective antagonist of glutamate's actions as discussed above, there are real concerns about chronic administration. Other glutamate antagonists have at least two well-documented adverse effects in the brains of people. First, they are neurotoxic and, with daily administrations, will eventually cause brain damage. Second, glutamate antagonists will reproduce many of the symptoms of schizophrenia in otherwise healthy people. In some cases, these symptoms do not fade away after drug use is terminated.

It can be argued that pyroglutamate is very safe since millions of people, by simply sticking to a balanced diet, take this amino acid every day without ill effect; pyroglutamate is in meats, dairy products, fruits, and vegetables. Unfortunately, this argument is not persuasive. There are many compounds found in low concentrations in food that, if isolated and given in higher doses, are toxic.

Typical doses
Doses of 500–1,000 mg per day are advertised by retailers. The basis for these dose levels is not known.

Contraindications
Pyroglutamate is contraindicated for people who are upset by the possibility of taking a drug for which there is little evidence of benefit and which may have significant risks. Due to the lack of trials of pyroglutamate in people, contraindicating medical conditions have not been identified.

The plain facts
Pyroglutamate has unproven benefits, unknown actions, and potential risks. Don't take this drug.

Benefits: 0
Risks: 5

TAURINE
Dietary supplement; available over the counter and through Internet suppliers

What is it?
Taurine is a sulfur-containing amino acid that is found in very high concentrations in the brains of all animals including humans.

Its reputation
Taurine is deemed the essential ingredient in drinks sold in Korea and China for the purpose of enhancing cognitive abilities.

The drug's effect on the brain
In addition to its presence in the brain, taurine is also found in high concentration in all living things including plants, algae, and all animals, where it has the same basic function: regulation and normalization of calcium levels inside cells. Although calcium is absolutely essential for the most basic operations performed by living cells that are necessary to sustain life, one of its most important roles is in the operations of the mitochondria, which, in turn, regulate energy levels. In addition, calcium is necessary to allow the release of neurotransmitters from neurons and is important in the regulation of excitability of all cells including neurons.

Taurine has been shown to be important for the normal development of infants' brains. Humans, unlike virtually all other animals, except cats, cannot synthesize taurine and are dependent on dietary sources of this amino acid. Although found in high concentrations in breast milk, taurine is not in sufficiently high concentrations in cow's milk. For this reason, it has been mandated that infant formula contains high levels of taurine.

It is also quite likely that this important amino acid is needed as we age. Moreover, it is also likely that the amounts of taurine that are derived from food are not sufficient for optimal functioning. The need for increased levels of taurine is based on the gradual decline of intracellular calcium levels, particularly in brain cells, in older people. With the decline in intracellular calcium is a concomitant decrease in the efficiency of the brain's energy metabolism, neuronal excitability, and neurotransmitter release.

How has it been tested? What are the risks, if any?
There are no studies of taurine's effects on cognition in people. In the 1970s, taurine was tested as a medication to decrease the frequency of epileptic seizures. Although effective for the first few months of administration, its beneficial influences on seizure activity gradually lessened as treatment continued. More recently, taurine has been used with positive results in several double-blind clinical trials testing efficacy in treating congestive heart failure. In its extensive use in both the epilepsy trials and in the congestive heart disease trials, taurine appeared to be virtually without risk of serious side effect. Indeed, only headaches were reported in a very small percentage of patients, and this adverse event was correlated with the use of extremely high doses. In large doses, taurine may be a depressant and actually impair short-term memory.

Typical dosages
Taurine, although well absorbed systemically, poorly penetrates the blood-brain barrier. Typical doses are therefore relatively high and usually 0.5–1 gram is taken daily.

Contraindications

Taurine has beneficial effects on patients with congestive heart failure, most probably through beneficial effects on the heart muscle's ability to contract. For this reason, persons with heart conditions characterized by increased excitability, such as certain arrhythmias, should consult their cardiologist before beginning taurine supplementation.

The plain facts

Taurine deserves our attention because of its unique and well-established physiological functions. An argument can be made for taurine supplementation based on the following factors:

- Neuronal calcium regulation is impaired with age.
- Efficient neuronal functioning is dependent on normal intraneuronal calcium.
- Taurine aids in the regulation of intracellular calcium levels.
- Humans must obtain taurine from their diet.
- Taurine appears to be without risk of serious side effects.

Unfortunately there is not one shred of scientific evidence from studies employing healthy humans that taurine has any effect on cognitive abilities. Taurine is included as an important ingredient in beverages sold in Korea and China and advertised to improve memory. However, only testimonials support the advertised claims.

Benefits: ½
Risks: 1

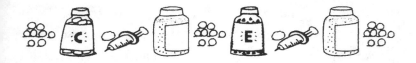

6

Hormones

In the first chapter of this book we discussed neurotransmitters, the chemical messengers that allow brain cells to communicate with each other. Neurotransmitters are produced in nerve cells and are released from nerve filaments (axon terminals) to float across the synapse and contact the immediately adjacent neuron. There is, however, a second type of chemical messenger that is also used by the body to allow different cells to communicate with each other. These substances, called hormones, are produced in endocrine glands (e.g., thyroid, adrenals, and ovaries) and secreted into the bloodstream, through which they travel to their targets. Unlike neurotransmitters that influence the immediately adjacent neuron, hormones often travel to quite distant destinations and they often affect many different areas. For example, thyroid hormone directly affects bone growth, liver function, the heart, the sympathetic nervous system, muscles, and the brain.

Physicians prescribe hormone supplementation to correct deficiencies due to disease; some smart drug advocates recommend certain hormones for healthy people to increase cognitive abilities. But unless there is disease, the body controls hormone levels very precisely so that momentary deficiencies or surpluses are corrected by adjustments in the rate of hormone synthesis and release. For virtually all hormones, concentrations above the body's normal level is as much a condition to be avoided as is a deficiency. Therefore, hormone supplementation in healthy people who are producing normal levels of hormones is not a good idea.

With aging, however, the output of many endocrine glands often decreases, with resulting decreases in hormone levels. Obvious examples are testosterone in males and estrogens in females. The secretions of these sex hormones usually drop precipitously as an individual approaches sixty years of age. Because hormones can influence the functioning of so many of the body's activities, it is possible that there could be effects on the brain's ability to function, which might be reflected by changes in memory, attention, and other cognitive processes. This chapter will review the evidence that hormone supplementation can increase cognitive abilities or restore declining powers brought about by aging and disease.

DHEA
Nonprescription hormone; available over the counter and through Internet suppliers

What is it?
DHEA (Dehydroepiandrosterone) is a hormone produced by the adrenals, small pyramid-shaped glands located on the upper tips of the kidneys.

Its reputation

Advocates of DHEA suggest that taking this hormone can, among many other benefits, reverse age-related memory loss and protect against neuron loss due to Alzheimer's disease. Based on their belief that the declining levels of this hormone in aging individuals is the cause of cognitive problems, some authorities advise attempting to restore DHEA levels to that of much younger individuals. This idea spawned a variety of studies in people on the effects of DHEA that suggest that using this hormone as a supplement may well be a double-edged sword.

DHEA's effect on the brain

Although DHEA itself is thought to have little biological action, it is converted by the body into a variety of other hormones such as estrogen and testosterone. However, this hormone is also synthesized in the brain by non-neural glial cells where DHEA has been shown to be capable of influencing the activity of receptors on neurons sensitive to various neurotransmitters. Thus, it is possible in theory for DHEA to influence thinking abilities either via the influences of testosterone and estrogen on brain activity or more directly by effects on the actions of neurotransmitters. It is possible—but does it actually have any effect?

How has it been tested? What are the risks, if any?

There is virtually no solid evidence indicating that DHEA use in young individuals has any beneficial effects. In contrast, a variety of studies support the notion of positive influences when DHEA administration is used in middle-aged to elderly persons to restore hormones to levels characteristic of younger individuals. Short-term (two weeks) use of DHEA, in double-blind, placebo-controlled trials, improves attention and information processing without any beneficial effect on memory. In another well-conducted study (double-blind placebo-controlled) of two-week administration, only the female subjects reported increased feelings of well-being and mood but no improvement in cognitive test results. Two double-blind placebo-controlled trials of longer administration (three months and six months) also reported improvements of feelings of well-being and, in addition, physical competence. With this more protracted hormone administration, both women and men reported similar psychological benefits. However, only men had measurable increases in muscle strength.

The fairly consistent reports of DHEA-induced increases in feelings of physical and mental well-being suggest the use of this hormone to treat depression. Indeed, one open study indicated that, in older depressed persons, use of DHEA could improve mood. This positive effect on mood could contribute to the anecdotal reports of DHEA-associated increases in cognitive functioning. Depression has a negative influence on many aspects of thinking including, most prominently, memory. In a depressed person, amelioration of affective problems would, secondarily, improve the ability to think.

Our review of the short-term and long-term trials of DHEA reveals no serious side effects; the most common adverse reaction appears to be acne. However, one shouldn't be sanguine about longer-term use of this hormone since six months seems to have been the most lengthy period of administration studied thus far. Consideration of DHEA's biological activities in the body underscores the need for caution; DHEA is converted to several important hormones, including the sex hormones estrogen and testosterone. Since estrogen and testosterone may stimulate the growth of several types of cancer in both women (breast, ovary, uterine) and men (prostate, testicular), persons with these diseases should not take DHEA. In addition, DHEA stimulates the production of insulin-like growth factor-I, a substance identified as a risk factor in cancer of the lung, breast, and prostate. DHEA can also interfere with pituitary and thyroid function.

Typical Dosages
In the majority of scientific studies of DHEA, a daily dose of 50 mg was used. However, daily doses as low as 30 mg and as high as 100 mg have been used.

Contraindications
DHEA is contraindicated for persons with cancer whether the disease is active or in remission. In addition, available evidence strongly suggests contraindication in persons with risk factors (e.g., family history or exposure to known carcinogens) for the development of cancer.

The plain facts
In summary, DHEA increases feelings of psychological and physical well-being that, in turn, can have beneficial effects on cognitive processes including memory. These advantages of DHEA must be weighed against a potential to exacerbate certain types of cancers and a risk, presently of undetermined magnitude, of increasing the chance of developing cancer.

Benefits: 3
Risks: 4

ESTROGEN
Hormone; available only by prescription

What is it?
Estrogens, female sex hormones, are primarily secreted by the ovaries in adult women. In addition, during pregnancy the placenta also secretes massive amounts. There are at least six estrogens although only three (beta estradiol, estrone, estriol) are present in significant concentration, with beta estradiol by far the most potent.

Its reputation
Until recently estrogen has primarily received attention from medical professionals, who are concerned with supplementation to stave off conditions such as bone loss, rather than consumers interested in this hormone's potential effect on cognition. However, reports that estrogens might delay the onset of Alzheimer's disease and/or have protective effects on mental functioning have stimulated more widespread interest. The idea that estrogens could improve memory is gaining currency in magazines, newspaper articles, and on the Internet, a trend that is only likely to increase.

Estrogen's effect on the brain
Estrogens are important for the development of the sexual organs and tissues, and they are also important in reproduction. In addition, estrogens influence skeletal growth, protein deposition, metabolism, hair distribution, and skin texture. More recently, estrogens have been demonstrated to enter the brain, where influences are exerted on neurotransmitters. This action could lead to possible consequences for cognitive processes.

How has it been tested? What are the risks, if any?
What are the consequences of the decrease of estrogen levels to almost zero following menopause? Examination of the effects of experimentally inducing a temporary menopause in younger women may provide part of the answer. Endometriosis is often treated by administering drugs such as leuprolide acetate (Lupron) that suppresses ovarian production of estrogens. Women receiving this drug report a variety of cognitive symptoms that most often include memory problems and depression. Most medical reports indicate that administration of beta estradiol in these patients reverses these symptoms. Is it therefore possible that increasing estrogen levels in postmenopausal women will also improve memory functions?

The evidence from clinical trials concerning estrogen's potential for improving cognitive functioning in postmenopausal women is not clear-cut. Studies of short-term administration do not strongly suggest any beneficial effects on cognitive test performance. In contrast, more protracted use of estrogen replacement does appear to improve memory, language abilities, and abstract reasoning. It may be significant that consistent across trials were reports of improved feelings of well-being associated with estrogen supplementation. Depression, a mental state that has negative effects on cognitive abilities, is associated with decreases in estrogen levels. It is conceivable that estrogen's ability to alleviate depression and its positive effects on mood contribute to or wholly underlie the beneficial effects of this hormone on cognitive abilities.

Is there a downside? Based on the available information, this question is difficult to answer. Numerous scientific papers have sought to determine if estrogen use in postmenopausal women increases risk of breast cancer. Studies conducted early in the 1990s suggest that there is indeed increased risk. More recent investigations are more reassuring, asserting that although there is some risk, it is slight. The small increase in the risk of breast cancer after long-term hormone replacement therapy use is likely to be outweighed by the positive effects of estrogens.

There can be, however, side effects that are not dangerous but should be taken into consideration when deciding whether or not to take estrogens. Most typical side effects include bloating, breast tenderness, and changes in mood.

Typical dosages

Estrogens are available in many different forms, and dosages further depend on which type of hormone is included and in what concentration. All are only obtained as prescription drugs and, if you are contemplating its use for cognitive enhancement, consultation with a physician is an absolute prerequisite.

Contraindications

Estrogens should not be taken in women with undiagnosed abnormal genital bleeding or who are pregnant or are suspected to be pregnant. Estrogens are also contraindicated for both men and women with known or suspected breast cancer or other estrogen-dependent neoplasias or a history of thromboembolic disorders or active thromboembolic disease.

The plain facts

Although the evidence is not clear-cut, it does appear that long-term use of estrogen replacement therapy does have a positive influence on memory, language abilities, and abstract reasoning. It is conceivable that these positive effects are brought about by estrogen's ability to alleviate depression. However, this must be weighed against studies that have shown that there is a slight risk of breast cancer after long-term hormone replacement therapy.

Benefits: 3
Risks: 1

GROWTH HORMONE

Prescription drug; available through a pharmacy and through Internet suppliers without prescription

What is it?

Growth hormone, also called somatotropin or somatotrophic hormone, is a small protein secreted by the pituitary that causes all living cells capable of growth to grow.

Its reputation

Growth hormone is promoted as a virtual fountain of youth that fights off the effects of aging. It is reputed to fix damaged cells, increase enzyme production, improve oxygen uptake, reduce the risk of stroke and heart attack, give your hair a healthy and youthful sheen, and, most important in the context of this book, generally improve cognitive functioning.

Growth hormone's effects on the brain

No definitive data or hypothesis has been advanced to explain why growth hormone supplementation should be of any benefit to healthy people. The shibboleth of many smart drug advocates, one that can be used as a rationale for taking scores of nostrums in the health food store, also applies to growth hormone. Specifically, growth hormone production decreases as we get older, so we need supplements. However, a specific effect of growth hormone on the brain that tends to diminish with age has not been identified. There are specific receptors for growth hormone located in many parts of the brain, including the hippocampus and cortex. Thus, circulating growth hormone does have some influence on brain cells. The nature of this influence, and whether it is of potential importance to any aspect of cognitive functioning, is not known.

How has it been tested? What are the risks, if any?
Growth hormone administration to laboratory rats improves learning ability, particularly in older animals. In humans, however, the picture is much less clear. There have been two double-blind studies of growth hormone's effects on cognitive processing in adults receiving supplementation due to hormonal deficiency. Although in the first study of nine patients, growth hormone improved mood, attention, verbal fluency, and other cognitive processes, in the second, larger study (forty patients) supplementation was without positive effect on any measure of cognitive functioning. In healthy elderly adults (fifty-two people, average age seventy-five years), a double-blind placebo-controlled trial failed to show any beneficial effect of growth hormone on cognitive functioning.

Growth hormone has only minimal risks for patients who are receiving supplementation under the control of a physician for the treatment of pituitary deficiencies. The most common adverse reaction is edema, which is seen in about 40 percent of patients. Unfortunately, little is known of the effects of growth hormone given to healthy people. Growth hormone can decrease the effectiveness of insulin so that patients with diabetes may require an adjustment of their therapy. Although growth hormone's ability to cause cancers has not been evaluated, the growth of certain preexisting cancers may be stimulated by this hormone. Acute overdose can induce hyperglycemia while chronic overdose can result in acromegaly (giantism in children). The symptoms and signs of acromegaly include swelling of the hands and feet, protrusion of the brows, lower jaw, and enlargement of the nose, carpal tunnel syndrome, deepening of the voice, excessive sweating, skin odor, fatigue, headaches, and, in men, impotence. The effects of acromegaly are diabetes mellitus, high blood pressure, and increased risk of heart disease and colon cancer.

Typical dosages
Growth hormone should only be taken under the guidance of a physician who will determine appropriate dosage.

Contraindications
Growth hormone is contraindicated in patients with cancer and should be stopped if cancer develops.

The plain facts
There is no convincing evidence that growth hormone supplementation in healthy adults had positive effects on memory, attention, or other aspects of cognitive functioning—and that's the plus side. On the minus side is risk of adverse reactions, some of which can make you both ugly and smelly and others of which can kill you. Does this sound like something you might want to take?

Benefits: 1
Risks: 4

PREGNENOLONE

Nonprescription drug; available over the counter and
through Internet suppliers

What is it?

Pregnenolone is a precursor in the synthesis of several important hormones. In plain English, pregnenolone, produced by
the body from cholesterol, is used as a building block to produce hormones such as DHEA (see discussion above), cortisol, and progesterone.

Its reputation

Pregnenolone is promoted as a powerful memory enhancer
that accomplishes this action by conversion to DHEA. It is
often combined with DHEA, reportedly to enhance the
effectiveness of DHEA.

Pregnenolone's effects on the brain

Smart drug advocates suggest that conversion to DHEA
underlies pregnenolone's advertised positive influences.
However, it is not clear whether pregnenolone, given to a
healthy individual, is necessarily converted to DHEA, rather
than progesterone, cortisol, or other hormones. If it is converted to cortisol, for example, pregnenolone would have
negative effects on learning and memory (see Chapter 2). It is
not even known if administration of pregnenolone necessarily
leads to increased production of any hormones at all.
Hormone production is very precisely controlled by the body;

unless there is a deficiency or disease, additional hormones are not synthesized even if there is an overabundance of precursors.

Pregnenolone also has the potential to produce effects by mechanisms that are independent of its role as a precursor to other hormones. Pregnenolone is known as a neurosteroid, a hormone that is independently produced in the brain by glial cells and that is able to modulate, or shape, the response of various receptors to certain neurotransmitters. There is evidence, for example, that pregnenolone can either enhance or suppress communication between neurons controlled by glutamate, the neurotransmitter that seems to be critical for learning.

How has it been tested? What are the risks, if any?
The effects of pregnenolone have been tested in numerous experiments with mice and rats, and it has been found to facilitate memory storage and enhance learning. In contrast, there have been no trials of pregnenolone's effects on cognitive processes in people.

Due to the lack of clinical trials, risks of pregnenolone can only be assumed. If converted to DHEA, all the risks associated with this hormone (see above) would also apply with pregnenolone. If converted to excess cortisol, there is a possibility of brain damage as well as toxicity when levels are high and withdrawal effects if drug administration stops and cortisol levels abruptly drop. These problems are complex and can be life threatening; discussion with a physician familiar with endocrinology should be undertaken before initiating pregnenolone administration.

High doses can cause insomnia, irritability, anxiety, acne, headaches, facial hair growth, loss of scalp hair, and heart rhythm irregularities.

Typical dosages

Suppliers furnish pregnenolone in 30, 50, and 100 mg capsules. There is no sound data on what constitutes either a reasonable or safe dosage, but some sources suggest that the daily dose not exceed 10 mg.

Contraindications

At the very least, the contraindications for DHEA also apply to pregnenolone.

The plain facts

There is absolutely no credible evidence that pregnenolone is of any benefit to cognitive processes in people. The risks of using this substance are similarly unclear though, if it is indeed converted to various hormones as advertised, there are potentially fatal side effects. The risk/benefit ratio is stacked strongly on the side of risk; taking pregnenolone is ill advised.

Benefits: 0

Risks: 4

VASOPRESSIN

Prescription drug: available through Internet suppliers

What is it?

Vasopressin—also called antidiuretic hormone (ADH), Ditressin, Syntopressin, and Diapid—is produced by neurons in an area called the hypothalamus and released by their nerve endings from the pituitary gland located at the base of the brain. Vasopressin is involved in regulation of water by acting on the kidneys to decrease the production of urine. Vasopressin, in high concentrations, can also cause contraction of smooth muscles (the type that form blood vessels, the gut, the bladder) and seems to act as a neurotransmitter in the brain.

Its reputation

Vasopressin is touted as a memory enhancer whose side effects can be annoying but are not dangerous. Misinterpreting some studies of vasopressin's effects in the brain, commercial suppliers include in their advertising copy statements to the effect that research has shown this hormone is *essential* to the ability to store memories.

Vasopressin's effect on the bra n

Although there is evidence that vasopressin is released by neurons in the brain, in addition to its release in the pituitary, its functions and effects are not known. Recent studies have suggested that very low concentrations of this hormone can facilitate the effects of the neurotransmitter glutamate while higher concentrations cause suppression. These effects are theoretically interesting since glutamate is thought to be critically involved in the first steps of memory storage.

Other studies have shown that vasopressin increases cortical activation. However, it is not known if this effect is due to a direct influence of vasopressin on the brain or this hormone's peripheral effects. Specifically, vasopressin can elevate blood pressure that, in turn, will increase arousal. It is possible that these activating effects rather than direct influences on the brain of vasopressin contribute to its effects on memory.

How has it been tested? What are the risks, if any?

Vasopressin or its analogues have been extensively tested on healthy young and old people as well as patients with a variety of disorders. It has been shown in several double-blind placebo-controlled trials that, in healthy young people, vasopressin had beneficial effects on memory. However, there is disagreement concerning whether the hormone's positive effects are exerted directly on memory or indirectly via improving attention. There is also some evidence that this hormone has stronger effects in males than in females. Two double-blind placebo-controlled trials demonstrated that vasopressin also improves memory processes in healthy elderly people.

The positive effects of vasopressin on cognitive processes in healthy young or older individuals is in contrast to its lack of efficacy in patients with a variety of disorders. Four double-blind placebo-controlled trials of vasopressin failed to find significant improvements in the cognitive functioning of patients with Alzheimer's disease or other forms of dementia. Other well-designed studies also found that vasopressin had no efficacy in treating memory or attentional impairments associated with schizophrenia, electroconvulsive therapy (ECT) in depression, or chronic alcoholism. The one exception found beneficial effects on memory and learning in children with attention deficit hyperactivity or learning disability.

Thus, vasopressin appears to be able to improve cognitive functioning in healthy people. However, there is an important caveat based on the nature of the positive trials. Although well designed, each of the positive trials studied very small numbers of people; the largest trial evaluated forty people. In addition, vasopressin was only administered for very short periods of time. The longest period of daily administration was three months; administration in the other trials varied from one to fourteen days. Because of the very small numbers of people tested and the short duration of treatment, the risks associated with vasopressin use in *healthy* people, particularly long-term use, are not known. For this reason, we should look to those people who take vasopressin for medical reasons to gain some idea of the potential risks.

Vasopressin, or its analogues, are prescribed regularly for the treatment of diabetes insipidus, a disease caused by the inability of the pituitary to release sufficient ADH. Because of this hormonal deficiency, patients with diabetes insipidus are unable to retain water and rapidly become dangerously dehydrated. Vasopressin is an effective treatment for patients with this disease who receive chronic hormone replacement therapy. The risks of administering too much vasopressin to such patients include cardiac arrhythmias, decreased cardiac output, and, less important, nausea, gastrointestinal cramping, flatulence, and the urge to defecate. In addition, vasopressin overdose can cause excessive retention of water, a condition known as hyponatremia or "water intoxication." In hyponatremia, excessive water retention leads to a dilution of the body's reserves of sodium, a metal that is critical for the most basic of the body's functions. The symptoms of water intoxication include lethargy, confusion, disorientation, and, if severe, seizures and coma.

Typical doses
Vasopressin or its analogues are given via nasal spray. Dosages depend on the particular analogue used and should be determined by consultation with a physician.

Contraindications
Vasopressin is contraindicated for people with kidney disease, heart problems (especially coronary artery disease), and primary or psychogenic polydipsia.

The plain facts

Several clinical trials indicate that vasopressin increases memory/attention in healthy people. In contrast, there are no indications that the use of this hormone is of any benefit to persons suffering cognitive problems due to Alzheimer's disease or other degenerative conditions. Despite its positive effects, the potential dangers of using this potent hormone outweigh the risks. Vasopressin can induce life-threatening complications with overuse in healthy people and, in persons with certain diseases (see Contraindications), even low doses can be fatal.

Benefits: 3
Risks: 5

One final point bears repeating with regard to the use of hormones in healthy people, that is, those without a hormonal deficiency. The human body employs many mechanisms that affect both the production of hormones and their release to ensure that specific concentrations are available. Hormone deficiencies cause significant symptoms and, as a result, are considered to be medical problems that require medical treatment (hormone supplementation). However, excess production of hormones also causes significant symptoms and is also properly considered to be a medical problem requiring medical treatment. When a healthy person takes hormone supplements, they are attempting to elevate hormone levels above normal and in effect induce a state that would ordinarily be considered to be a medical problem. To a certain extent, the body will compensate for the excess hormone due to supplementation by reducing its own production of that hormone. However, it is possible to override the body's natural protective mechanisms and induce a hyper-hormonal condition. It must be recognized, however, that this condition is no different from the excess hormonal states associated with many diseases and, like those illnesses, is associated with significant medical symptoms.

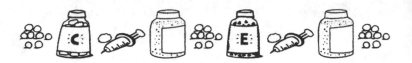

7

Vitamins

A vitamin is defined as an organic (carbon-containing) molecule, that cannot be produced by the body but is necessary for normal functioning. There are probably hundreds of such compounds although at present only a small number have been identified. While there are minimum amounts of each vitamin required for adequate health, the actual measure necessary differs for a given individual as a function of several variables. For example, during periods of growth, greater amounts of certain vitamins are needed. They are also needed during pregnancy, nursing, and disease. To metabolize large amounts of carbohydrates, one's intake of thiamine and other B vitamins should be increased. Unfortunately, we can only estimate the minimum required amounts, and for many vitamins there have been protracted debates concerning where to draw the line. For example, beginning in the 1970s, Nobel laureate Linus Pauling argued strenuously that the typical intake of vitamin C was woefully short of what the body actually required for normal functioning. Interestingly, this debate continues to the present.

Since the body cannot manufacture vitamins, a person

must obtain these important substances through diet or by vitamin supplements. Because diets differ, as do requirements for specific vitamins, deficiencies in specific areas can easily occur. Hints that vitamins may play an important role in cognitive functioning primarily come from studies of the symptoms suffered by people with various deficiencies. For example, it has been repeatedly shown that the level of cognitive functioning of geriatric patients correlates with their history of vitamin supplementation. Unfortunately such investigations do not necessarily prove a causal role for vitamin deficiencies in cognitive deficits; people with cognitive impairments may have poor nutrition as a result of deficient thinking rather than the converse. More definitive evidence for a role of vitamins in cognitive functioning has been recently provided by both a clearer understanding of how individual vitamins work and also by better designed trials using human subjects.

NIACIN
Dietary supplement; available over the counter and through Internet suppliers

What is it?
Niacin, also called vitamin B_3 or nicotinic acid, functions in the body when converted to nicotinamide adenine dinucleotide, an enzyme important in tissue respiration. Large doses of niacin are sometimes used to treat high levels of cholesterol.

Its reputation
Niacin or its analogues are promoted as memory boosters that are effective in healthy young and middle-aged people.

Several advertisements stress niacin's ability to increase blood flow to the brain.

Niacin's effect on the brain

Niacin's principle effects on the brain are most probably exerted via its important role in tissue respiration. There is no convincing evidence that niacin increases cerebral blood flow, has specific effects on any neurotransmitters or their receptors, is either neuroprotective or neurotrophic. However, there are some indications, although not definitive, that xanthinol nicotinate, a niacin derivative, does increase circulation and improve cerebral metabolism.

How has it been tested? What are the risks, if any?

Several double-blind placebo-controlled trials of niacin's influences on patients with various types of dementia (e.g., Alzheimer's disease, multi-infarct dementia) have shown that this vitamin improves cognitive functioning and may slow the rate of deterioration. Xanthinol nicotinate, possibly a more effective derivative of niacin, was also shown in double-blind placebo-controlled trials to improve cognitive functioning of patients with various types of dementia.

One interesting double-blind placebo-controlled trial compared the efficacy of niacin to xanthinol nicotinate in healthy people. Each was administered to persons in three age groups: "young" (35–45 years of age), "middle aged" (55–65 years) and "old" (75–85 years). Niacin improved the ability of members of the young and middle-aged groups to process information and also enhanced their short-term memory. In contrast, xanthinol nicotinate was more effective with older people and not only enhanced information processing and short-term memory but also improved long-term memory.

The adverse reactions to niacin include flushing of the face, extreme itchiness, gastrointestinal distress (pain, nausea, vomiting, diarrhea), and, more significantly, peptic ulcers and toxic effects on the liver. The latter effects are most often seen with the megadoses of niacin (2–6 grams per day) that are sometimes used to treat elevated cholesterol levels. Facial flushing is most often seen at the initiation of chronic treatment and decreases with repeated administrations. Niacin or its derivatives may interact with drugs taken to treat hypertension and enhance their effects potentially resulting in dangerously low blood pressure. There is also a suggestion that niacin may exacerbate cardiac arrthymias.

Typical dosages

In the clinical trials, the dosages varied depending on whether niacin or one of its derivatives were used. For example, niacin was administered in the range of 141 mg, nicergoline 20 mg, and xanthinol nicotinate at 1–3 grams. All clinical trials tested daily dosing lasting two to three months.

Contraindications

Niacin and related drugs are contraindicated for patients with liver disease, cardiac arrhythmias, and either ulcer disease or a propensity to develop ulcers. Significant interactions with antihypertensive medications are also possible.

The plain facts

Niacin and related compounds have beneficial effects on cognitive functioning of healthy people and also those with impairments due to various forms of senility. In the absence of contraindicated conditions, these compounds also appear to be relatively safe.

Benefits: 4

Risks: 1

PYRIDOXINE
Dietary supplement; available over the counter and through Internet suppliers

What is it?
Pyridoxine, vitamin B_6, is a water-soluble molecule that is involved in the metabolism of several amino acids that are important for bodily functions, including the formation of several of the brain's neurotransmitters. In addition, B_6 also influences the actions of other hormones in the body by modulating the receptors to which these hormones ordinarily attach.

Its reputation
Pyridoxine is advertised as a way to "boost intelligence," improve memory, learning, and possibly, to enhance creativity. In addition, pyridoxine is suggested to have these beneficial effects without either toxic side effects or addictive potential.

Pyridoxine's effect on the brain
B_6 is clearly important for the normal functioning of the brain since persons with deficient intake of this vitamin suffer seizures as well as inflammation of peripheral nerves. B_6 deficiencies are also characterized by abnormally lowered concentrations of amino acid neurotransmitters.

How has it been tested? What are the risks, if any?
In view of the effects of B_6 on neurotransmitters, it is not surprising that the actions of this vitamin also appear to affect
cognitive processes. In a one-year double-blind placebo-
controlled trial, healthy young adults were given a supplement
consisting of nine vitamins at ten times the recommended
daily allowance. Both males and females reported improvements in mood when on the supplement as compared to periods when on the placebo. Further analysis showed that this
mood change was most closely associated with riboflavin and
B_6 levels in the blood. Other work also suggests that B_6 has
positive effects on mood. There are several clinical reports
describing the efficacy of B_6 supplementation as a treatment
for depression suffered by women taking oral contraceptives.
It should be noted that positive effects on emotional state
could, in depressed individuals, result in improvements in
overall cognitive functioning.

In a three-month placebo-controlled trial of B_6 administration to elderly men, significant improvements in memory
storage were observed. In this study, moderate doses of B_6
were used. In a second trial, doses five to fifty times higher
were tested using a similar experimental design. In contrast to
the beneficial effects of moderate doses, high doses of vitamin B_6 significantly impaired memory.

The amount of pyridoxine required increases with dietary
protein intake. For every 100 grams of protein in the diet, at
least 1.5 mg of B_6 is needed. Based on the typical diet of U.S.
citizens, if such a diet actually exists, the FDA has estimated
that the required daily allowance of B_6 for adults should be
1.6 mg for women and 2 mg for men. Good sources of B_6
include meat, liver, soybeans, and vegetables.

There are several potential dangers of which the potential

user of vitamin B$_6$ must be aware. First, consumption of large daily doses of pyridoxine (200 mg/day) results in neurotoxicity. Second, there have been reports that use of large daily doses can produce symptoms of dependence. Third, B$_6$ supplementation reduces the effectiveness of drugs taken to alleviate the symptoms of Parkinson's disease.

Typical dosages

The RDA for pyridoxine is 1.6 mg for women and 2 mg for men. Dosages ten times these levels are typically used in scientific studies of the cognitive effects of pyridoxine and 50 mg is customarily prescribed, without ill effect, for the treatment of carpal tunnel syndrome. In contrast, doses as high as 200 mg are to be avoided since these drug levels are clearly toxic to nerve cells.

Contraindications

Pyridoxine reduces the effectiveness of L-DOPA, a drug that is commonly used to treat Parkinson's disease and also, on occasion, restless leg syndrome. Patients taking L-DOPA should consult with their neurologist before starting pyridoxine supplementation to discuss the advisability of this course of action and the possibility of compensatory adjustments in the dosage of L-DOPA.

The plain facts

Studies have shown that pyridoxine (vitamin B$_6$) supplementation in moderate amounts under 2 mg a day have resulted in measurable improvements in memory storage and emotional states. However, large daily dosages (200 mg per day) of pyridoxine carry significant risks, such as neurotoxicity, symptoms of dependence, and a reduction in the efficacy of drugs for Parkinson's disease.

Benefits: 4
Risks: 2

THIAMINE
Dietary supplement; available over the counter and through Internet suppliers

---

What is it?
Thiamine, also known as vitamin B_1, enables the body to metabolize carbohydrates and use them for energy.

Its reputation
Curiously, thiamine has no significant reputation among smart drug enthusiasts. It has, however, been noted for its antioxidant properties.

Thiamine's effect on the brain
Because metabolism of carbohydrates is the primary source of energy for brain cells, thiamine deficiency can have extremely deleterious effects on brain functioning. It is therefore both interesting and perplexing that this critical vitamin has received virtually no attention from the advocates of smart drugs.

How has it been tested? What are the risks, if any?
Thiamine supplementation is quite safe since, as a water-soluble vitamin, excess thiamine is excreted. Foods rich in

thiamine include pork, organ meats, legumes, and nuts. The required daily allowance (RDA) of this vitamin increases with carbohydrate intake. Moreover, older people appear to require increasing levels of thiamine. Because this vitamin is not well stored in the body, changes in diet or physiological requirements can quickly lead to thiamine deficiency. For example, caffeinated tea and certain species of raw fish that can be eaten as sushi contain chemicals that break down thiamine or block its actions in the body. Consuming large amounts of these foods can result in a temporary deficiency.

Long-term (twelve months) administration of a mix of ten vitamins (one of which was thiamine), at ten times the recommended dose, was used with young healthy adults in a double-blind placebo-controlled trial. Cognitive testing showed that females only demonstrated a significant improvement in attention. Analysis of vitamin concentrations in the blood revealed that this beneficial effect of supplementation was correlated specifically with increases in thiamine levels. In a second placebo-controlled study, the same group of scientists showed that two months of thiamine supplementation led to self-perceived feelings of being "more clear-headed, composed and energetic." In addition, subjects receiving thiamine showed significantly better reaction times.

Thiamine has also been used to treat cognitive disorders associated with disease. One open study reported improvements in emotional and cognitive functioning of mildly impaired Alzheimer's patients after receiving a thiamine derivative. More convincing, a double-blind placebo-controlled trial with thiamine in moderately impaired Alzheimer's patients showed a significant improvement in overall cognitive functioning. Finally, a double-blind placebo-controlled trial of thiamine in abstinent former cocaine abusers showed that vitamin supplementation improved their impaired memory functioning.

Typical dosages
The recommended daily dietary (RDA) allowance of thiamine, established by the Food and Nutrition Board of the American Academy of Sciences is shown in the table below:

RDA in Mg for Thiamine			
Age	11–14	15–50	51+
Male	1.3	1.5	1.2
Female	1.1	1.1	1.1

In many of the scientific studies of the cognitive effects of thiamine, ten times the RDA was used without ill effect.

Contraindications
There are no contraindications for the use of thiamine.

The plain facts
In summary, thiamine is a safe vitamin with actions critical to the normal functioning of the brain. Since the RDA of thiamine is dependent on many variables, it is worthwhile to carefully evaluate your needs and, if necessary, take a dietary supplement.

Benefits: 4
Risks: 0

VITAMIN B$_{12}$

Dietary supplement; available over the counter and through Internet suppliers

What is it?

Vitamin B$_{12}$, also known as cyanocobalamin or simply cobalamin, is essential for the replication of DNA and is therefore intrinsic to cell growth and division.

Its reputation

B$_{12}$ has a strong reputation as a general heath tonic or revitalizer and has been specifically recommended to fight off age-related decreases in cognition in general and memory in particular.

B$_{12}$'s effect on the brain

B$_{12}$ is critical for the normal development of the brain and is involved in a variety of processes during growth, including covering nerve fibers with myelin, a fatty sheath that facilitates the ability of neurons to conduct electrochemical activity. B$_{12}$ also facilitates the activity of glutamate, an excitatory transmitter that is thought to be central to the brain's capacity to learn from experience and to store information. In addition, B$_{12}$'s importance to brain functioning can also be seen in the consequences of deficiencies. Loss of the myelin sheaths, the covering of axons, occurs in both the brain and in nerves that are involved in the sense of touch and vision. In addition, with prolonged deficiency neurons die throughout the brain. The symptoms of nervous system damage with B$_{12}$ deficiency include loss of the sense of touch, movement problems, memory loss, confusion, and psychosis.

How has it been tested? What are the risks, if any?

People obtain B_{12} from food; this vitamin is in highest concentration in animal products and, to a lesser extent, in legumes. However, the most common cause of B_{12} deficiency is not inadequate diet, but rather an inability to absorb B_{12}, a problem that is fairly uncommon in younger people but shows increasing incidence with advancing age. Frequently, a B_{12} deficiency is detected, not as a cognitive problem, but through the appearance of the most obvious symptom of inadequate levels of B_{12}, pernicious anemia. Blood cells have a very short life span and, as a result, there is an unremitting need to generate new cells. Since B_{12} is critical for the replication of DNA and therefore intrinsic to cell growth and division, lack of this vitamin impairs the production of new blood cells.

Given B_{12}'s renowned reputation as a general tonic and memory booster, it is surprising that search of the medical literature revealed no solid trials in which supplementation was tested in persons without vitamin deficiencies. Consequently, there is no reliable information concerning B_{12}'s potential for affecting cognitive functioning in healthy people. Conversely, B_{12} has been tested extensively in people with cognitive impairment and demonstrable B_{12} deficiency. In such cases, B_{12} supplementation frequently results in amelioration of impairments, provided that deficiency hasn't persisted so long that permanent brain damage has resulted.

It is not advisable, however, to attempt to treat an apparent B_{12} deficiency, particularly if detected due to anemia, by taking multivitamin supplements without the guidance of a physician. For reasons whose explanation is beyond the scope of this book, B_{12} deficiency results in a lack of ability to use another essential vitamin, folic acid. Folic acid, like B_{12}, is critical for the generation of new blood cells. Most multivitamins contain, in addition to B_{12}, folic acid. The levels of folic acid in many multivitamins are typically sufficient to compensate for the lack of B_{12} with respect to the growth of new blood cells while B_{12} levels in these supplements may not be high enough to restore that vitamin to normal levels. Taking such a multivitamin can, by curing the anemia, give the erroneous impression that the vitamin deficiency has been fixed. However, since the B_{12} deficiency in fact persists, damage to the brain will continue.

Typical dosages

The recommended daily allowance (RDA) of vitamin B_{12} is 2 μg per day.

Contraindications

There are no known contraindications.

The plain facts

Although vitamin B_{12} is essential for the normal functioning of the brain, the effects of supplementation in people without a B_{12} deficiency are not known. In contrast, B_{12} often, but not always, improves the cognitive functioning of people with impairments due to deficiencies. In the event of insufficient B_{12}, a program of therapy should be worked out by a treating physician.

Benefits: 1
Risks: 1

VITAMIN E

Dietary supplement; available over the counter and through
Internet suppliers

What is it?

Vitamin E, also known as alpha-tocopherol, is a fat-soluble
vitamin with known antioxidant properties.

Its reputation

Vitamin E is promoted as an antiaging vitamin and frequently included as an ingredient in formulations that also
contain smart drugs, herbs, and other vitamins and are advertised as either brain energizers or memory enhancers.

Vitamin E's effect on the brain

While specific effects of vitamin E on the brain have not
been described, the effects of a lack of this vitamin are well
known. In laboratory animals fed a vitamin E deficient diet,
degeneration of nerve fibers in various parts of the brain
occurs as well as accentuated brain injury from exposure to
certain toxins. In people who lack the ability to absorb vitamin E, problems develop that affect the ability to walk normally and the sense of touch.

How has it been tested? What are the risks, if any?

There is very little known of the effects of vitamin E supplementation in humans. A recent study of over four thousand
people, sixty years and older, showed a correlation between
low intake of vitamin E and memory problems. There was no
correlation between memory problems and deficiencies of
vitamins A or C. The researchers acknowledged a difficulty
of interpretation in that it was not clear if "low (blood) levels

of vitamin E preceded the onset of poor memory or that low levels of vitamin E are a result of having poor memory."*

Vitamin E also has been tested in Alzheimer's disease. The rationale for its use is that death of neurons in this disease is caused in part by the deposit of beta-amyloid in plaques. Beta-amyloid achieves its toxic effects in part through oxidative stress. Hence, an antioxidant such as vitamin E should, in theory, slow the progress of this disorder. A large double-blind placebo-controlled trial evaluated the effectiveness of vitamin E and found that supplementation did indeed slow progression in moderately impaired patients.

Typical dosages

Sufficient vitamin E is present in almost any human diet to supply the RDA (15/12 IU). In the clinical trial described previously, 2,000 IU were administered daily for two years.

Contraindications

Patients taking anticoagulants should avoid high doses of vitamin E, which could enhance the effects of these medications. Iron should not be taken with vitamin E, since the absorption of both could be diminished. Those suffering from diabetes, rheumatic heart disease, an overactive thyroid, or high blood pressure should not use high doses.

The plain facts

According to the available evidence, vitamin E is essential for normal brain function and deficiencies may cause memory problems. A normal diet and perhaps supplementation with

*from Health Central
http://www.healthcentral.com/news/newsfulltext.cfm?ID=13747

an appropriate multivitamin should be all that is necessary to supply sufficient vitamin E for healthy people. The evidence for vitamin E supplementation for Alzheimer's patients is promising though, at this point, only one study has been performed.

Benefits: 2
Risks: 0

Only those vitamins that have been generally recommended, or, in the case of pyridoxine, *should* have been recommended to improve cognitive functioning were discussed in the previous paragraphs. However, it should be recognized that deficiencies of other vitamins, including riboflavin, pantothenic acid, biotin, and vitamin C, can negatively impact the functioning of the nervous system. Many studies indicate that distressingly high percentages of people in the United States have diets deficient in at least one important vitamin. Moreover, the older we get, the more likely it is that we will have a vitamin deficiency. Not only do our likes and dislikes often result in an unbalanced choice of foods, we are also more likely either to have diseases that can decrease vitamin absorption or to be taking medicines that can have such an effect. It is for this reason that, if you believe that you are beginning to experience cognitive problems, consideration of your diet is definitely a prudent course of action.

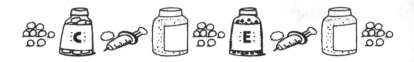

8

Oxygen

Although some organisms on this planet have evolved to thrive in environments where there is little or no oxygen, this is not the case with humans. We are *aerobic* creatures; i.e., we require oxygen for every process of life and when we are deprived of oxygen even for a short period of time, our body organs suffer the consequences. The brain is perhaps the organ most sensitive to the effects of oxygen deprivation. This is probably due to the high energy demands of the functioning brain. Thus, only a few minutes of oxygen deprivation can have catastrophic consequences on the brain. But, while oxygen is essential for the normal functioning of brain cells (and just about every other cell in our bodies), too much oxygen is not necessarily a good thing. In fact, there are a number of potentially dangerous chemicals called reactive oxygen species that are singularly associated with life as an oxygen-consuming creature. Some of these reactive oxygen species can be formed as the normal by-products of certain physiological processes in our bodies while others are produced only under pathological conditions. Regardless of how they are produced, reactive oxygen species are potentially very dangerous. For instance, these chemicals have the ability to damage DNA, alter cellular proteins necessary for normal functioning, and ultimately to cause cell death. Thus, it is an ironic paradox that the very oxygen that is absolutely necessary to sustain our aerobic lives can also initiate the formation of potentially harmful compounds that can destroy living cells.

Reactive oxygen species can either be a class of chemicals called radicals (such as the hydroxyl radical or the superoxide radical) or can be nonradical compounds that easily enter into chemical reactions such as singlet molecular oxygen and hydrogen peroxide. Some of these reactive oxygen species, particularly the hydroxyl radical, can react instantly with neighboring molecules (DNA, RNA, lipids, proteins) causing oxidative damage to cells. There are many sources of reactive oxygen species in living organs, including the human brain. One common source, for example, is the metabolic breakdown of certain neurotransmitters (see Chapter 3 for discussion of neurotransmitters). When the neurotransmitter dopamine is metabolized or broken down, free radicals and hydrogen peroxide are generated. Under normal circumstances, our brains contain efficient enzyme and antioxidant systems that neutralize these potentially damaging chemicals before they have a chance to harm our cells. There is normally a delicate balance between reactive oxygen species formation and antioxidant defense mechanisms. However, in certain disease conditions, antioxidant defenses become overwhelmed and certain nerve cells may become abnormally sensitive to the production of free radicals and related compounds. Under these circumstances, cells enter a state of "oxidative stress" that may make these nerve cells vulnerable to destruction. Oxidative stress can be produced by a number of internal and external factors such as genetic makeup and exposure to toxins. Oxidative stress, left unchecked, is one of the processes involved in damaging cells in a variety of disorders from Parkinson's and Alzheimer's diseases to cancers.

Although the use of oxygen in medicine has a long history, the application of oxygen-based treatments for the amelioration of cognitive problems is much more recent and controversial. A variety of oxygen therapies are regularly used, from the familiar oxygen mask/tent to the more esoteric hyperbaric oxygen chamber to the absurd liquid oxygen drinks. Oxygen mask/tent and hyperbaric oxygen chambers are forms of treatment that have accepted uses in clinical medicine. Oxygen is routinely administered in hospitals, hospices, and in homes to persons having difficulty breathing due to a variety of diseases. Hyperbaric therapy, in which a person breathes 100 percent oxygen while under heightened barometric pressure to increase absorption, is traditionally used to treat injury from radiation, healing-resistant wounds, crush injury, carbon monoxide poisoning, and other conditions that can be ameliorated by increasing exposure to oxygen. The use of hyperbaric oxygen to enhance mental abilities is not an accepted application of this treatment.

The rationale for using oxygen therapies to increase cognitive powers or to counteract age-related memory loss is based on the theories that under normal conditions cells do not get as much oxygen as they need and that, as a person grows older, oxygen does not reach a person's brain in sufficient concentration to sustain normal functioning. There is absolutely no scientific evidence that any of these conditions occur with any frequency. "Oxygen bars" have opened in several major cities where the public is told that they can wake up their brains with a whiff of pure oxygen from a pressurized tank. Potential customers are told that oxygen therapy is needed to replenish depleted oxygen in their systems and that it allows the body to direct oxygen to its primary functions without having to draw on valuable reserves. Assuming that you are a healthy person who is breathing on a regular basis and that your blood contains a normal number of functioning red blood cells, there should be no reason why you should experience oxygen depletion. Also, holding your breath is probably the only way for you to maintain (at least a short-term) a reserve of oxygen in your body. Some individuals go to oxygen clinics where they are sealed in a hyperbaric chamber for treatment at about $200 per hour. Besides the hour of solitude that this provides (which in and of itself may be therapeutic for some of us) does this or any of the other oxygen-related products actually improve mental powers, and are they safe?

OXYGEN THERAPY

What is it?
Oxygen is a colorless, odorless gas that is part of the air we breathe and the water we drink. All cells in our bodies, and particularly cells in our brains, require oxygen for survival.

Its reputation
Oxygen therapy is the inhalation of pure oxygen. Professional athletes inhale pure oxygen before and during competition to boost their energy levels. Promoters of oxygen therapy claim that inhaling pure oxygen can increase mental performance and alertness. Oxygen therapy is becoming increasingly popular in trendy locations known as oxygen bars where patrons can inhale pure or "flavored" oxygen.

Oxygen's effect on the brain

Oxygen is vital to normal cell functioning and is the fuel for all cellular activities. Irreversible brain damage and death of nerve cells can occur rapidly after loss of oxygen (blood flow) to the brain. Most of the presumed benefits of oxygen therapy, including increased energy and vigilance, come from anecdotal reports and testimonials.

How has it been tested? What are the risks, if any?

There is very little data in the scientific literature that shows that excess oxygen or pure oxygen improves cognitive performance. One double-blind placebo-controlled study using twenty subjects showed that breathing pure oxygen improved performance on a simple word recall task in healthy young adults while breathing normal air had no effect on performance. In addition, oxygen administration improved performance on several measures of attention and vigilance. Oxygen therapy had no effect on other aspects of cognitive performance, including spatial memory and memory of numbers, and no effect on mood. While the merits of oxygen therapy in healthy individuals are still a matter of debate, oxygen therapy may have beneficial effects in the treatment of cluster headaches and specialized hyperbaric oxygen therapy may have use in the treatment of certain types of traumatic head injuries.

Although oxygen is vital to life, it is possible to have too much of a good thing. Many experts argue that there is no reason for a healthy individual to require extra or pure oxygen. In fact, a healthy individual living at or near sea level has about as much oxygen contained in his or her blood as it is capable of storing. Pure oxygen, if breathed for prolonged periods, can become toxic. Oxygen can poison nerve cells when the dose and duration of exposure are sufficient. Too much pure oxygen may cause release of excessive amounts of potentially toxic oxygen free radicals, which can irreversibly damage nerve cells. Signs of oxygen toxicity are irregularity in breathing patterns, twitching, dizziness, and in extreme cases, seizures.

Typical dosages

Oxygen therapy uses 100 percent oxygen; dose is varied by manipulating exposure time. Typically 20–30 minutes is the maximum exposure used.

Contraindications

1. Long exposure time: Ordinarily twenty-four hours of continuous exposure to pure oxygen is deemed toxic, although it should be noted that this figure was determined for people with lung disease in which inflammation and mucus afforded the lung tissue some protection from the damaging potential of pure oxygen. It is possible that the maximal allowable exposure of normal people would be shorter than twenty-four hours, though it is not known how much shorter. On the other hand, it is highly unlikely that the typical exposure time in oxygen bars, less than thirty minutes, would be harmful to healthy people.

2. People with emphysema: A subset of such patients will experience breathing difficulties of life-threatening severity if exposed to pure oxygen.

The plain facts

Oxygen therapy or inhaling pure oxygen may produce some short-lived improvements in very limited types of cognitive functions. It will not cause general improvements in cognitive functioning and has no direct effect on mood. In small doses, it is unlikely to do any real harm. Prolonged or excessive use of pure oxygen can have detrimental effects on nerve cells.

HYPERBARIC OXYGEN THERAPY

What is it?

"Hyper" means increased and "baric" means pressure. Hyperbaric oxygen therapy involves intermittent treatment of the entire body with 100 percent oxygen at above normal atmospheric pressures. Hyperbaric oxygen therapy increases oxygen concentration in all body tissues, may stimulate the growth of new blood vessels into areas with reduced circulation, and aids the treatment of infection by enhancing the action of germ-fighting white blood cells.

Its reputation

Hyberbaric oxygen therapy is touted as a treatment of chronic degenerative health problems related to atherosclerosis, senility, peripheral vascular disease, and other circulatory disorders. It is also used for treatment of healing-resistant wounds and has recently gained attention for its use in children with cerebral palsy. The recognized indications for the use of hyperbaric oxygen are:

Gas embolism
Carbon monoxide poisoning
Decompression sickness
Clostridial myonecronsis (gas gangrene)
Selected wound problems

Severe anemias
Necrotizing infections (flesh-eating bacteria)
Osteomyelitis
Radiation tissue damage
Compromising skin grafts
Thermal burns
Intracranial abscess
Diabetic sores

Hyberbaric oxygen's effect on the brain

Although hyperbaric oxygen may have effects on brain capillaries, there are no scientific reports of the effects of hyperbaric oxygen on brain function or activity in normal individuals. Most of the presumed benefits of hyperbaric oxygen therapy come from anecdotal reports and testimonials.

How has it been tested? What are the risks, if any?

A number of animal studies have examined the effects of hyperbaric oxygen on the brain. While some studies claim that hyperbaric oxygen initiates cellular and vascular repair processes after certain types of brain injury, other studies have not found this to be the case. On the contrary, some studies have found that exposure to hyperbaric oxygen can cause formation of reactive oxygen species and cause damage to cells. In general, animal studies seem to suggest that exposure to hyperbaric oxygen, up to about two atmospheres of pressure, does not result in oxygen toxicity to nerve cells, but that may change with exposure to pressures of much greater than two atmospheres. There have been no animal studies of the effects of hyperbaric oxygen on cognitive functioning. However, one study did examine the effects of exposure to hyperbaric oxygen on cerebral circulation and the oxygen supply to the brain in rats. The main finding of this study was that the oxygen supply to the brain was essentially unchanged during breathing of hyperbaric oxygen.

A search of the MEDLINE database did not produce any scientific articles on the effects of breathing hyperbaric oxygen on cognitive functions in normal young or elderly people. However, there have been some studies of the effects of hyperbaric oxygen on brain function in impaired populations. In patients suffering from carbon monoxide poisoning of moderate severity, hyperbaric oxygen treatment was reported to improve short-term recall for word lists. However, in another study of carbon monoxide–poisoned individuals, normal cognitive functions were reported at one year follow-up with or without the use of hyperbaric oxygen. Hyperbaric oxygen therapy has also been attempted on elderly patients with vascular dementia, on patients with acute ischemic stroke, and on elderly patients with "organic brain damage" and cognitive impairment of unknown origin. In the majority of these studies, no significant changes in cognitive functioning were reported in association with hyperbaric oxygen therapy. More than four hundred cases of human ischemic stroke treated with hyperbaric oxygen have been reported. In about one half of these cases, improvement in cognitive status has been claimed. Yet, due to various flaws and confounds in the conduct of many of these clinical studies, there is no clear-cut evidence to either support or refute the potential benefits of hyperbaric oxygen therapy for elderly patients with organic brain damage of mixed etiology.

The risks associated with repeated use of hyperbaric oxygen are similar to the risks associated with breathing pure oxygen. If the pressure of the hyperbaric oxygen is not carefully controlled, there is the risk of generation of oxygen toxicity, development of seizures, and permanent brain damage.

Typical dosages

Typical hyperbaric oxygen therapy used for defined medical purposes uses oxygen at 2–2.5 atmospheres pressure. Typically about thirty minutes is the maximum exposure used.

Contraindications

Similar as for the use of pure oxygen.

The plain facts

There is no evidence that hyperbaric oxygen therapy yields improvements in any types of cognitive functions in normal healthy individuals. At properly regulated doses, it is unlikely to do any real harm. However, prolonged or excessive use of hyperbaric oxygen can have detrimental effects on nerve cells.

LIQUID OXYGEN THERAPY

What is it?

Liquid oxygen (LOX) is perhaps best known as a fuel for liquid-fueled rockets. Although the oxygen around us exists as a gas, if air is cooled enough, it will change from a gas into a liquid or a solid. Oxygen turns to a liquid at −183 degrees Celsius.

Its reputation

Other than its reputation as an oxidizer in liquid-fueled rockets or as a source of gaseous oxygen (it takes up a lot less space to store compressed liquid oxygen in tanks than to store oxygen gas) it essentially has no real health-related uses.

Some unscrupulous retailers are trying to sell products billed as "stabilized liquid oxygen" as a "rich supply of dissolved and bio-available stabilized oxygen" to replace oxygen lost in our bodies due to "toxic stress, emotional stress, physical trauma and infections, reduction in available atmospheric oxygen [not a common occurrence on this planet], improper diets and lack of exercise." These products are nothing more than water with oxygen bubbled through it. Such hyper-oxygenated waters are worthless products since water can only contain so much oxygen no matter how much extra oxygen you try to pump into it. Even if you can hyper-oxygenate water, the excess oxygen is lost to the air very quickly.

How has it been tested? What are the risks, if any?
No research has been done on the effects of hyper-oxygenated water on cognitive functioning, and we can't think of anyone who would even think to try to use real liquid oxygen (remember it's kept at −183 degrees Celsius) for anything other than rocket fuel. Basically, this stuff is nonsense and it will most likely have no positive effects on any cognitive processes. However, if you feel compelled to try one of these liquid oxygen drinks, probably the only negative effect it will have is on your wallet.

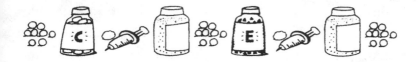

9

What's in the Research Pipeline?

Neuroscience, the scientific study of the brain, has undergone unprecedented growth in the past twenty years. This expansion was spurred, in part, by remarkable advances in genetics, molecular biology, and computer technology as well as a presidential proclamation and joint resolution of both houses of Congress designating the 1990s as the "Decade of the Brain." The "Decade of the Brain" resolution proposed to increase public awareness and legislative support of brain research and, for the most part, has lived up to its promise. Neuroscience is now one of the fastest growing areas of science in the United States, as illustrated by the recent meeting of the Society for Neuroscience at which over twenty thousand neuroscientists presented reports describing new results from their laboratories.

Important advances have been made in many areas, including identification of the factors that control the growth, survival, and repair of neurons; clarification of the ways in which the brain "learns" and stores or "remembers" information; and descriptions of the chemical reactions and neural circuits involved in the performance of many of the brain's activities. Based on these discoveries, unique chemical compounds are being synthesized in the laboratory with the purpose of affecting the brain chemistry, structure, and function and, in so doing, altering behavior. It is highly probable that some of these drugs will eventually make their way into general use as smart drugs and/or medications to lessen the cognitive impact of some neurodegenerative diseases. This chapter will discuss some of the new approaches currently being developed in the lab and the purposes for which new therapeutic agents might be used in the future.

Neuroprotective Agents

Although brain cells are delicate and highly vulnerable to a variety of stimuli that adversely affect their survival, ultimately neurons almost always die in one of two ways: apoptosis or necrosis. Apoptosis, also known as programmed cell death, is a process in which the neuron, in essence, commits suicide. This type of cell death occurs when a neuron is exposed to some extreme stressor that sends a message to the neuron's genes to trigger a series of reactions in that cell that have the purpose of shutting down all life-sustaining activities. Normally, apoptosis takes place during development when extra brain cells are eliminated through a genetically controlled pruning and culling process. In fact, the beautifully orchestrated sculpting process that takes place during the maturation of the human brain results in the loss of about half of all neurons born during neurogenesis. Neurons are thought to compete for precious resources such as growth and survival factors secreted in the brain and as in other aspects of life, it's survival of the fittest. Those neurons that are less successful in making proper connections with other neurons do not receive an adequate supply of growth and survival factors and subsequently die. In mature brains, apoptotic cell death may be involved in neuron death in diseases such as Alzheimer's and Parkinson's.

The second way in which neurons die is through necrosis. Necrosis ensues when neurons are exposed to some trauma or toxin that causes cellular processes (such as respiration and energy production) compatible with life to cease. Necrotic neurons often look different than neurons undergoing apoptosis. In apoptosis, the cell usually begins to die through disruption of the genetic machinery housed in the nucleus. In necrosis, the cell usually begins to die through disruption of internal organelles such as mitochondria (the cell's energy factory) and endoplasmic reticulum (where proteins are made and transported).

One of the major contributing factors to neuronal cell death is excitotoxicity, the demise of one neuron at the "hands" of another neuron. Excitotoxicity is caused when one neuron releases an excitatory neurotransmitter called glutamate. Under ordinary conditions, the effect of glutamate at the synapse is simply to activate an adjacent neuron. However, under pathological conditions, an excess amount of glutamate released into the brain can overexcite adjacent neurons and cause their death. Excitotoxic cell death occurs during a variety of neurodegenerative diseases and also during brain injury from trauma, anoxia (lack of oxygen), and ischemia (decreased blood flow). Because synaptic transmission involving glutamate lies at the heart of excitotoxic cell death, it is possible to prevent this pathological process by blocking the actions of glutamate. Drugs that block glutamate's effects are called neuroprotective agents. More generally, neuroprotective drugs can protect against any of a variety of causes of cell death and in theory might be helpful in treating stroke, anoxia, traumatic brain injury, and a variety of neurodegenerative diseases. A number of such drugs are being tested in laboratories around the world although none of them, because of a variety of problems, should be in general use anytime soon.

Glutamate Receptor Blockers

One potent blocker of glutamate's activities is phencyclidine, also known as PCP, or Angel Dust. Unfortunately, this drug's side effects, including schizophrenia-like symptoms and brain damage, do little to recommend clinical usefulness. There are a number of other neuroprotective agents being tested, including dizocilpine (MK-801), ketamine, and dextromethorphan, which, because of their own sets of side effects, cannot be used in human patients. However, the use of glutamate blockers as neuroprotective medications holds promise for the future and, when safer agents are developed, will have uses in the treatment of many diseases and conditions that compromise brain functioning.

GM1 Ganglioside

Gangliosides are chemicals that are abundantly present in the outer covering of neurons called the cell membrane. Neurons communicate with each other by releasing chemicals that contact specialized receptors located in the cell membranes. In addition, hormones affect the activity of neurons by entering the brain through the circulation and contacting receptors in the cell membranes. Because of their integral place in the cell membrane, gangliosides play important roles in cell signaling and modulate the way cells respond to different types of messages. There are many types of gangliosides. The ganglioside that currently appears most promising is called GM1 ganglioside. It plays an important role in a number of cell functions and is involved in the transfer of information from outside of the cell to the interior of the cell. GM1 seems to enhance the production of certain neurotrophic factors and can enhance the way cells respond to neurotrophic factors. Unlike neuroprotective agents that block glutamate's toxic effects, GM1 ganglioside seems to help damaged neurons to repair themselves.

GM1 ganglioside has been tested in both laboratory animals and in clinical trials involving people. Numerous studies in animals have shown GM1 to reverse age-related deficits in memory and to reduce the effects of various types of injury on the nervous system. Numerous well-conducted studies have shown that GM1 ganglioside can protect against certain types of brain injury and, in other instances, can stimulate the injured brain to repair itself after injury. Despite a plethora of positive findings from animal studies, there have only been a few well-conducted human clinical trials with GM1. In one study, GM1 was found to significantly improve motor and cognitive functioning in Parkinson's disease patients. Another study showed that long-term use of GM1 could slow the progression of symptoms in Parkinson's disease patients. Other studies have shown positive effects in stroke patients and significant improvements in sensory and motor functioning in people with acute spinal cord injury. Alzheimer's disease patients who received GM1 ganglioside infused directly into their brains were found to have modest improvements in various activities of daily living. The available data show that GM1 ganglioside is very safe. No clinically significant adverse effects have been noted with continued use of this drug, in some cases, up to four years. Administration of excessively high doses (2,000 mg/day) results in temporary elevation of cholesterol and triglyceride levels that return to normal when GM1 administration is stopped. Currently, this drug is only available in an injectable form. It is not approved for any clinical use in the United States, but it is currently used in South America as a treatment for stroke, diabetic neuropathy, and Parkinson's disease.

Neurotrophic Factors

Neurotrophic factors are naturally occurring chemicals that support growth and survival of neurons. While neurotrophic factors are important during the development of the nervous system, they also appear to play important roles in the maintenance of neuronal connections and neuronal functioning in the adult nervous system. In some neurodegenerative disorders, it is believed that a loss of trophic support underlies the death of specific types of neurons. Thus, therapies have been attempted in which neurotrophic factors are administered in an attempt to stop cell death or cause regrowth of damaged neurons.

While the theory of neurotrophic factor therapy is sound, in practice it has not worked well. First, it is very difficult to get neurotrophic factors into the brain; they do not readily cross the blood-brain barrier, a natural barrier system designed to keep certain types of substances out of the brain. Second, neurotrophic factors are not specific for a single neuronal type, so it has proven very difficult to affect only the desired type of neurons without also having effects on other types of neurons. Nonetheless, studies in animals have shown that administration of a particular neurotrophic factor, nerve growth factor, delivered directly into the brain, can ameliorate some of the neurochemical and behavioral problems associated with experimentally produced syndromes that resemble Alzheimer's disease. Neurotrophic factor therapies (nerve growth factor, brain derived neurotrophic factor, glial cell derived neurotrophic factor, fibroblast growth factors, ciliary neurotrophic factor, and insulin-like growth factors, to name a few) are continuing to be developed, and if their current shortcomings can be overcome, they hold promise to be effective agents in the fight against a variety of neurological disorders.

Ampakines

Glutamate is an amino acid that acts as an excitatory neurotransmitter and is found in high concentrations throughout the brain. Although glutamate is involved in many processes, it has been extensively implicated in learning and memory. Ampakines are a group of compounds that act on a type of glutamate receptor called the AMPA receptor. When these compounds bind to this receptor, they cause excitation of the neuron. Ampakines or drugs that bind to the AMPA receptor hold the receptor open longer than glutamate itself, enhancing the excitation of the neurons and supposedly contributing to the memory-enhancing capabilities of these drugs. Ampakines have been touted as memory enhancers, primarily from work performed in animals. Based on findings of enhanced memory in rats, at least one ampakine, AMPALEX, has been tested in humans. In a double-blind placebo-controlled study involving twenty-four healthy volunteers, the AMPALEX group performed better on some tests of learning and memory in comparison to people who received placebo. The drug appeared safe, although it was only administered over a five-day period, and long-term safety data are lacking. Nonetheless, ampakines represent a potential new therapy for certain cognitive and memory disturbances, and their future development will have to be watched closely.

Xanthine Derivatives

Xanthine derivatives are a class of drugs with varied functions including vasodilation (i.e., increasing blood flow), reduction of free radicals, and stimulation of synthesis of nerve growth factor. In addition, these drugs increase the activities of adenosine, a neurotransmitter with effects in many areas of the brain. One such xanthine derivative, propentofylline, has been shown to prevent degeneration of acetylcholine-containing neurons in rat models of stroke and Alzheimer's disease and to improve memory functions in treated animals. Propentofylline has been assessed in humans in patients with ischemic stroke, Alzheimer's disease, and vascular dementia (dementia due to impaired blood flow to the brain). One placebo-controlled trial using propentofylline and four using a related drug, pentoxifylline, were conducted using almost eight hundred people. There were no significant effects on death rates and data on neurological impairment and disability were inconclusive. Data on quality of life were not reported. Propentofylline in the treatment of Alzheimer's disease and vascular dementia have reached the Phase III stage of testing. Nine hundred and one patients with mild/moderate Alzheimer's disease and 359 patients with mild/moderate vascular dementia were enrolled in four double-blind placebo-controlled trials ranging in duration from six to thirteen months. Consistent improvements over placebo in efficacy assessments have been found for both patient groups. Other data also suggest that in addition to relieving some of the dementia symptoms of Alzheimer's disease, propentofylline may slow the progression of impairments. The drug appears to be safe and well tolerated. This drug has not been tested for possible cognitive-enhancing effects on nondemented people.

Gene Therapies

Gene therapies hold promise to ameliorate the effects of many of humankind's health problems. Cures or treatment for devastating diseases like cancer may be amenable to therapies where faulty or missing genes are replaced. Such therapies are no longer science fiction but science reality. Can gene therapy be used to improve cognition? According to one scientist from Princeton University, the answer is yes. In the laboratory, mice were bred to have extra copies of a subtype of a special glutamate receptor called the NR2B subunit of the NMDA receptor. The NMDA receptor has long been known to be involved in memory processes. With extra amounts of this NR2B receptor, mice were claimed to be "smarter" and have better memory than their compatriots with only the usual amount of NR2B receptors. This was touted in the media as a finding that could boost human intelligence and this new strain of mice were actually dubbed "Doogie" after the precocious young genius doctor on the television series *Doogie Howser, M.D.* But does improvement on tests of spatial learning and memory and better performance on other learning and memory tests in mice really suggest anything about the potential for gene therapy to boost human intelligence? The answer is no. Human intelligence is much more than simple learning and memory of spatial concepts, and there is no way to equate performance of mice in the lab with human intelligence. Does gene therapy of the type just discussed hold promise as a way to reverse human memory deficits? Perhaps. Even if such therapies could improve deficient memory, expecting such therapies to improve normal memory is another thing altogether. For the time being, genetically enhanced memory in mice is an interesting and enticing finding, but the excitement must be tempered with the reality that we are entering areas here in which we have a very thin base of knowledge on which to build.

Index

abstract thinking and reasoning:
  aging and, 51
  hormones and, 39, 173–75
  moods and, 37
  smart drugs and, 68
acetylcholine:
  amino acids and, 162
  future therapeutic agents and, 220
  smart drugs and, 72–74, 84–87,
    98, 110, 118–19, 131, 135, 139,
    141, 144, 147, 149
acetylcholinesterase inhibitors, 86–87,
  118
acetylcholinesterases, 118
acetyl-l-carnitine, 153–56
acromegaly, 177
adaptogens, 109
adenosine, 79, 220
ADH (antidiuretic hormone)
  (Ditressin) (Syntopressin)
  (Diapid) (vasopressin), 180–84
adrafinil (Olmifon), 69–72
adrenal glands, 37, 40, 69, 127, 168
adrenaline (epinephrine), 69, 103,
  127–28
age, aging, 50–52
  amino acids and, 153–54, 156,
    159, 161–62, 165–66
  concentration and, 15–17
  future therapeutic agents and, 217
  genetics and, 44–45
  hormones and, 168–70, 173,
    175–76, 181–82

  information and, 82
  lifestyle changes and, 52
  medical problems of, 51–52
  memory and, 12–13, 15–17, 45,
    51–52, 65, 88–89, 91, 95, 106,
    124, 137, 139, 144, 154, 156,
    161, 169, 187–89, 191, 196,
    199, 204, 217
  oxygen and, 204, 210
  smart drugs and, 81–82, 88–91,
    94–95, 98, 100–103, 106–7,
    110, 113, 115, 123–24, 132,
    135, 137, 139–40, 143–44
  vitamins and, 187–89, 191,
    194–97, 199, 201
alcohol, alcoholism, 33
  amino acids and, 153–55, 161
  hormones and, 182
  memory and, 62–63
  negative influences of, 49–50
alertness, 21
  oxygen and, 205
  smart drugs and, 79–80, 121
allergies, 14, 49
alpha-adrenergic agonists, 69–71
alpha-glycerylphosphoryl-choline
  (alpha-GPC), 72–74
alpha-tocopherol (vitamin E),
  199–201
aluminum, 40–41, 43–44
Alzheimer's disease:
  aluminum and, 43–44
  amino acids and, 153–58, 160–61

Alzheimer's disease (cont.)
future therapeutic agents and, 215,
217, 219–20
genetics and, 45–46
hormones and, 169, 172, 182, 184
and negative influences of drugs, 48
oxygen and, 204
smart drugs and, 73–75, 84–90, 93,
99–100, 102, 105–8, 118–22,
125–26, 135, 137–38, 142, 144,
147–48
and testing drugs and dietary supplements, 35
vitamins and, 188, 194–95, 200–201
American Academy of Sciences, Food
and Nutrition Board of the, 195
American ginseng, 109, 111
American Pharmaceutical Association,
17
American Society of
Anesthesiologists, 14
amino acids, 25, 152–66
future therapeutic agents and,
215–17, 219, 221
side effects of, 155–56, 165–66
smart drugs and, 75, 118–19, 125,
131, 139, 141, 157, 159
vitamins and, 190, 196
see also specific amino acids
amnesia, 61
ampakines, 219–20
AMPALEX, 219
amphetamines, 50, 69, 92, 100
androgens, 38–39
androstenedione, 39
anemia, 24, 197–98
Angel Dust (phencyclidine) (PCP),
216
animal testing, 27–30
aluminum and, 43
amino acids and, 154, 162
future therapeutic agents and,
217–21
genetics and, 46
hormones and, 176, 179
MSG and, 43
oxygen and, 209–10
smart drugs and, 70, 72–73, 75, 78,
82, 88, 91, 93, 98, 110, 119–20,
125, 132, 135, 139, 142, 144,
146–47
vitamins and, 199
see also mice; monkeys; rats
aniracetam, 74–77, 136, 144
antibiotics, 22, 51
anticoagulants, 33, 107–8, 111, 117,
140, 150
anticonvulsants, 94
antidepressants, 11, 33, 93
human testing of, 30–31
negative influences of, 47
smart drugs and, 103–4
antidiuretic hormone (ADH)
(Ditressin) (Syntopressin)
(Diapid) (vasopressin), 180–84
antiemetics, 134
antihypertensives, 51, 89, 133
anti-inflammatories, 51, 142
NSAIDs and, 47–48, 129
smart drugs and, 106–7, 118
antioxidants:
negative influences of, 48
oxygen and, 203
smart drugs and, 78, 81–82, 90, 93,
102, 106–7, 110, 113–14,
124–26
vitamins and, 193, 199–200
aplastic anemia, 24
apolipoprotein E (APO-E), 44–45
apoptosis, 214–15
Asian ginseng, 109, 111
aspirin, 11, 29, 33, 107, 140, 142, 150
negative influences of, 47–48
Attentil (BP662) (Visilor) (fipexide),
100–102
attention:
amino acids and, 153–55, 157, 159
hormones and, 39, 168, 176–77,
182, 184
and influence of moods on brain,
37
memory and, 63–64
and negative influences of drugs,
47, 50
oxygen and, 206
smart drugs and, 68, 69–70, 73,
90–91, 101, 109, 111, 133, 137,
140, 146–47

and testing drugs and dietary supplements, 28
attention deficit hyperactivity, 64, 182
Avan (Tap) (idebenone), 124–26
axons, 54–55
    amino acids and, 154
    and drugs in improving thinking, 64
    information and, 57–58
    smart drugs and, 127, 135
    vitamins and, 196
axon terminals, 54, 56, 118, 167

back pain, 11–12
bacopa (brahmi) (water hyssop), 77–79
bacterial infections, 22
barbiturates, 33
beta amyloid, 154, 200
beta blockers, 51, 89, 133
beta estradiol, 172–73
Big Blue, 53
biotin, 201
birth control pills, 92–93, 191
blood clotting, 14
    anticoagulants and, 33, 107–8, 111,
    117, 140, 150
    smart drugs and, 107–8, 116–17,
    140, 150
bones, hormones and, 167, 172
BP662 (Visilor) (fipexide) (Attentil),
    100–102
brain:
    comparisons between computer
    and, 36, 60
    effects of body chemistry on, 38–40
    injuries to, 61–62, 64, 75, 87–88,
    132, 145, 199, 206, 209–10,
    216–17

caffeine, 69, 79–81, 115–16
calcium, 25
    amino acids and, 164–66
    smart drugs and, 94–95, 149
calcium channel blockers, 78, 129–34
cancers, 14
    children and, 41
    future therapeutic agents and, 221
    hormones and, 171, 174–75, 177
    oxygen and, 204
    smart drugs and, 80, 113, 116

cats, 29
Cavinton (vinpocetine), 148–51
CDP-choline (cytidine 5'-diphospho-
    choline) (citicoline), 87–89
Centella asiatica (Indian pennywort)
    (*Hydrocotyle asiatica*) (talepe-
    trako) (gotu kola), 112–14
Centers for Disease Control, 34
centrophenoxine (Lucidril), 81–83
cerebellum, 49, 61
Charney, Dennis, 30–31
children, 17, 40, 64
    amino acids and, 164–65
    cancers in, 41
    hormones and, 177, 182
    smart drugs and, 95, 99, 143
Chinese restaurant syndrome, 40,
    42–43
cholesterol, 178, 218
    vitamins and, 187, 189
choline, 21, 72, 84–87, 98
citicoline (cytidine 5'-diphospho-
    choline) (CDP-choline), 87–89
clarity:
    smart drugs and, 70, 77
    vitamins and, 194
cocaine, 69, 195
    negative influences of, 49–50
coenzyme Q-10, 124
cognitive functioning, 34–35
    see also specific mental processes
concentration, 21
    amino acids and, 159
    effects of age on, 15–17
    and impact of moods on brain, 37
    smart drugs and, 94, 118, 121, 146
    and testing drugs and dietary sup-
    plements, 30
concept formation, 30
Congress, U.S., 14, 213
control groups:
    animal testing and, 28
    in human testing, 30–32
    see also double-blind placebo-
    controlled trials; single-blind
    placebo-controlled trials
cortex:
    hormones and, 176
    smart drugs and, 72–73, 144

cortisol (hydrocortisone), 40, 140
178–79
Coumadin (warfarin), 33, 107–8, 111,
117, 140, 150
Crapper-McLachlan, Donald, 43
creativity:
smart drugs and, 141
vitamins and, 190
cyanocobalamin (vitamin B_{12}), 196–98
cytidine 5'-diphosphocholine (CDP-
choline) (citicoline), 87–89

Dean, W., 112, 127n, 133
deanol (DMAE) (dimethyl-
aminoethanol), 81, 98–100
Decade of the Brain resolution, 213
declarative memory, 62–63
dehydroepiandrosterone (DHEA),
168–71, 178–80
dementia:
amino acids and, 161
future therapeutic agents and, 220
genetics and, 45
hormones and, 182
smart drugs and, 76, 82–83, 107,
122, 132–35, 137–38
vitamins and, 188
dendrites (somas), 54–56
deprenyl (selegiline hydrochloride)
(Eldepryl), 89–93
depression, 11
amino acids and, 153, 155, 165
hormones and, 170, 173, 175, 182
impact on brain of, 37–38, 40, 51
and negative influences of drugs, 47
smart drugs and, 103, 113, 133
vitamins and, 191
see also antidepressants
deoxyribonucleic acid (DNA), 45
neurons and, 54
oxygen and, 203
vitamins and, 196–97
dextromethorphan, 216
DHEA (dehydroepiandrosterone),
168–71, 178–80
diabetes, 177, 183
Diapid (vasopressin) (antidiuretic hormone) (ADH) (Ditressin)
(Syntopressin), 180–84

Dietary Supplement Health and
Education Act (DSHEA), 14, 25
dietary supplements, 22–35, 67
deaths caused by, 33
definition of, 25
differences between drugs and,
25–27, 34
effectiveness of, 25–29, 31
evaluating risk of, see risk/benefit
ratios
interactions of, 14, 33
side effects of, 11–12, 14, 26, 32
standardization of ingredients of, 34
testing of, 23–24, 26–32, 34–35
digoxin, 111
Dilantin (phenytoin), 94–97
dimethylaminoethanol (DMAE)
(deanol), 81, 98–100
disorientation, 51
and negative influences of drugs, 49
smart drugs and, 90
Ditressin (Syntopressin) (Diapid)
(vasopressin) (antidiuretic hormone) (ADH), 180–84
dizocilpine (MK-801), 216
DNA, see deoxyribonucleic acid
Doctor's Always In, The (Lidsky and
Schneider), 18
dopamine:
oxygen and, 203
Parkinson's disease and, 64–66
smart drugs and, 70–71, 79, 87, 90,
92, 100–101, 103, 131, 139,
144, 192
double-blind placebo-controlled trials,
31–32
amino acids and, 154–55, 158–59,
162, 165
future therapeutic agents and,
219–20
hormones and, 170, 176, 182
on MSG, 42–43
oxygen and, 206
smart drugs and, 73, 75–76, 80, 82,
85–86, 88, 91, 95, 99, 101,
103–4, 106, 110–11, 113, 115,
119, 122–23, 125, 128, 132–33,
135, 137, 140, 142–44, 147,
149–50

vitamins and, 188, 191, 194–95, 200
double-blind trials, 31–32
Down's syndrome, 45, 153, 155
drug, drugs, 12–14, 61–62
    aging brain and, 51–52
    after approval, 24
    average cost of development of, 24
    deaths caused by, 26, 33
    definition of, 22
    differences between dietary supplements and, 25–27, 34
    effectiveness and risks of, 21–35
    in future, 216
    how they have their effects, 64–67
    interactions of, 14–15, 22, 33, 51
    negative influences of, 46–50
    prices of, 13
    side effects of, 12, 22–24, 26
    standardization of ingredients of, 34
    testing of, 23–24, 26–32, 34–35
DSHEA (Dietary Supplement Health and Education Act), 14, 25
dyslexia, 143

Ecstasy, 50
education, 45–46
Eldepryl (selegiline hydrochloride) (deprenyl), 89–93
electromagnetic waves (electrical fields), 40–42
emotions, see depression; moods; specific emotions
emphysema, 207
endocrine glands, 167–68
energy:
    amino acids and, 153–54, 164–65
    oxygen and, 202, 205
    smart drugs and, 79, 81, 87, 109, 118, 124
    vitamins and, 193–94
enkephalins, 100–101
environment, 44–46
eosinophilia, 101
epilepsy, 24, 33, 61
    amino acids and, 165
    oxygen and, 207, 210
    smart drugs and, 77, 82–83, 94–96, 104, 113

vitamins and, 190
epinephrine (adrenaline), 69, 103, 127–28
episodic memory, 62–63
ergoloid mesylates (Hydergine), 120–24
ergot, 120–21
estrogens, 92, 168–69, 171–75
    impact on brain of, 38–39
etiracetam, 136, 144
excitatory neurotransmitters, 57, 59
    amino acids and, 162
    future therapeutic agents and, 215, 219
    smart drugs and, 118
    vitamins and, 196
excitotoxicity:
    amino acids and, 160
    future therapeutic agents and, 215
    smart drugs and, 119, 131–32, 134
executive functioning:
    amino acids and, 154–55
    and negative influences of drugs, 49
    smart drugs and, 80
    and testing drugs and dietary supplements, 28
expectorants, 33
experimental groups:
    animal testing and, 28
    human testing and, 30–32

fats (lipids), 138–39, 203
Federal Food, Drug, and Cosmetic Act, 22
Felbatol, 24
fetus development, 17
fipexide (Attentil) (BP662) (Visilor), 100–102
folic acid, 25, 197–98
Food and Drug Administration (FDA), 14–15, 67
    on dietary supplements, 25
    drugs regulated by, 22, 24, 26–27, 34
    smart drugs and, 137–38
    vitamins and, 191
forgetfulness, see memory
free radicals, 220
    amino acids and, 153
    oxygen and, 203, 207

free radicals (cont.)
   smart drugs and, 75–76, 81–82, 90,
      93, 99, 106–7, 110, 121–22,
      124–26
frontal lobe, 59, 61
functional magnetic resonance imaging (functional MRI), 60–61
future therapeutic agents, 213–22

gamma-aminobutyric acid (GABA),
   73, 131, 144, 152
garlic, 14
gene therapies, 221–22
genetics, 44–46
   future therapeutic agents and,
      213–15
   oxygen and, 203–4
gerovital (GH–3), 102–4
ginger, 14
gingko biloba, 13–14, 105–8
ginseng, 14, 109–12
glial cells, 179, 219
glucocorticoids, 37–38, 40
glutamate, glutamates, 152, 157, 162–63
   future therapeutic agents and,
      215–17, 219, 221
   hormones and, 179, 181
   smart drugs and, 75, 118–19, 125,
      131, 139
   vitamins and, 196
glutamate receptor blockers, 216
glycine, 156–58, 160
GM1 ganglioside, 216–18
gotu kola (Centella asiatica) (Indian
   pennywort) (Hydrocotyle
   asiatica) (talepetrako), 112–14
grapefruit juice, 33
grapes, 26
growth hormone (somatotropin)
   (somatotrophic hormone),
   175–78
guarana (Paullinia cupana), 115–17

hallucinations, 92
haloperidol, 129
heart, heart problems, 14, 33, 49,
   165–67
   aging brain and, 51–52
   amino acids and, 165–66

hormones and, 167, 175, 177, 179,
   183
   smart drugs and, 71, 80, 92, 102,
      104, 109–10, 112–13, 116–17,
      127, 129, 132–34, 147
   vitamins and, 189
hemorrhaging, see blood clotting
herbs, herbal remedies, 25
   from China, 34
   government on, 14–15
   risks and benefits of, 11–15
high blood pressure, see hypertension
hippocampus, 38, 49
   hormones and, 176
   information and, 59–61
   smart drugs and, 72–73, 144
homeopathic preparations, 15
hormone replacement therapy, 174–75,
   183
hormones, 37–40, 69, 167–85
   future therapeutic agents and, 216
   impact on brain of, 38–40
   memory and, 39–40, 63, 168–75,
      177–79, 181–82, 184
   moods and, 37
   sex, 38–39, 92, 168–69, 171–75
   side effects of, 170, 174, 176,
      180–81
   vitamins and, 190
human testing:
   amino acids and, 154–55, 158–59,
      162, 165
   of drugs, 23–24, 26–32
   future therapeutic agents and, 217,
      219–20
   hormones and, 170, 173, 176, 179,
      181–84
   on MSG, 42–43
   oxygen and, 206
   placebo-controlled trials in, see
      double-blind placebo-controlled
      trials; single-blind placebo-
      controlled trials
   smart drugs and, 70–71, 73, 75–76,
      80, 82–83, 85–86, 88, 90, 95,
      99, 101–4, 106, 110–11, 113,
      119, 122–23, 125, 128, 132–33,
      135, 137, 140, 142–45, 147,
      149–50

vitamins and, 188–89, 191, 194–95, 197, 199–200
huperzine A *(Huperzia serrata)*, 117–20
Hydergine (ergoloid mesylates), 120–24
hydrocortisone (cortisol), 40, 140, 178–79
Hydrocotyle asiatica (Indian pennywort) (*Centella asiatica*) (talepetrako) (gotu kola), 112–14
hydrogen peroxide, 203
hydroxyl radicals, 203
hyperbaric oxygen therapy, 204–6, 208–11
hyper-oxygenated waters, 212
hypertension, 14, 33, 49, 51, 133
  smart drugs and, 71, 80, 83, 89, 93, 102, 104, 109, 112, 126–27
  vitamins and, 189
hypotension:
  smart drugs and, 88–89, 91–92, 102, 104, 109, 128–29
  vitamins and, 189
hypothalamus, 180
hypoxia, 76, 98

ibuprofen, 11, 47, 129
idebenone (Avan) (Tap), 124–26
Inderal (propranalol hydrochloride), 126–30
Indian pennywort (*Centella asiatica*) (*Hydrocotyle asiatica*) (talepetrako) (gotu kola), 112–14
information, 57–64
  aquisition and retrieval of, 51
  and drugs in improving thinking, 64
  integration of, 58–59
  neurons and, 57–60, 64, 82
  processing of, 80, 91, 95, 188–89
  storage of, 59–64, 153, 158, 196, 213–14
  transfer of, 82, 217
inhibitory neurotransmitters, 57, 59
insomnia, *see* sleep, sleep problems
insulin, 177
intelligence quotients (IQs), 61
  genetics and, 44
  smart drugs and, 94–95
Internet, 17–18, 22
ischemia, 75

Kasparov, Garry, 53
kava kava, 14–15, 33
Kefauver-Harris Drug Amendments, 22
Kessler, David A., 24
ketamine, 216
kidneys, kidney problems, 14, 81, 153
  hormones and, 180, 183

language ability, *see* verbal fluency
L-DOPA, 65–66, 192
lead, lead poisoning, 34, 41
learning, 42
  amino acids and, 154, 157, 162
  attention and, 64
  future therapeutic agents and, 213–14, 219, 221
  hormones and, 176, 178–79, 182
  and impact of moods on brain, 38
  information and, 60
  MSG and, 43
  and negative influences of drugs, 49–50
  smart drugs and, 73, 75, 78, 82, 84, 88, 95, 100, 109, 112, 115, 119–20, 125, 132, 135, 139, 141–42, 146–47
  and testing drugs and dietary supplements, 28–29, 32
  vitamins and, 190, 196
lecithin, 84–87
leukemia, 41
leuprolide acetate (Lupron), 173
Li Chung Yon, 113
lifestyle changes, 52
lipids (fats), 138–39, 203
lipofuscin, 82
liquid oxygen (LOX) therapy, 211–12
liver, 14, 33
  amino acids and, 153, 159–60
  hormones and, 167
  smart drugs and, 96, 101, 125, 129, 136
lobelia, 33
locus coeruleus, 146
long-term memory, 62–63
  smart drugs and, 142
  vitamins and, 189
low blood pressure, *see* hypotension

Lucidril (centrophenoxine), 81–83
lysergic acid diethylamide (LSD), 121

McGwire, Mark, 39
Magnetic Resonance Imaging (MRI),
    42, 60–61
MAO (monoamine oxidase), 103
marijuana, 49–50
MEDLINE, 70, 91, 149, 210
MedWatch, 24
memory, 21
    aging and, 12–13, 15–17, 45,
        51–52, 65, 88–89, 91, 95, 106,
        124, 137, 139, 144, 154, 156,
        161, 169, 187–89, 191, 196,
        199, 204, 217
    amino acids and, 153–59, 161–62,
        165
    and drugs in improving thinking,
        64–65
    future therapeutic agents and,
        213–14, 217, 219–22
    genetics and, 45
    hormones and, 39–40, 63, 168–75,
        177–79, 181–82, 184
    influences on, 37–40, 47, 49–50,
        63–64
    information and, 59–64
    moods and, 37–38, 63
    MSG and, 43
    oxygen and, 204, 206, 210
    smart drugs and, 68, 70, 72–77, 80,
        82, 84–85, 87–91, 95, 101,
        105–9, 112–13, 115, 118–21,
        124, 128–33, 135–48, 150
    and testing drugs and dietary sup-
        plements, 28, 30, 32, 34–35
    types of, see specific types of memory
    vitamins and, 187–92, 195–97,
        199–201
menopause, 39, 173–74
menstrual cramps, 34
messenger ribonucleic acid (RNA), 60
methamphetamine, 92
mice:
    amino acids and, 154
    future therapeutic agents and, 221
    hormones and, 179
    smart drugs and, 70, 110, 112, 142

testing drugs and dietary supple-
    ments on, 29
Milacemide, 156–61
mitochondria, 153, 156, 164, 215
MK-801 (dizocilpine), 216
monkeys:
    smart drugs and, 70, 119
    testing drugs and dietary supple-
        ments on, 29
monoamine oxidase (MAO), 103
monosodium glutamate (MSG), 40,
    42–43
mood disorders, 49, 99
    see also depression
moods:
    hormones and, 170, 173–74, 176
    impact on brain of, 37–38, 40, 51
    memory and, 37–38, 63
    oxygen and, 206, 212
    smart drugs and, 101
    vitamins and, 191–92, 194
Morganthaler, J., 112, 127n, 133
morphine, 26
MRI (Magnetic Resonance Imaging),
    42, 60–61
muscles, muscle relaxants, 33, 42
    hormones and, 167, 170, 181
myelin, 196

narcolepsy, 69
National Library of Medicine, 70
natural solutions, equating good with,
    13
nature/nurture, 44
necrosis, 214–15
nervous system, 201
    future therapeutic agents and,
        217–18
    hormones and, 167
neural tube defects, 25
Neuroactiv (Neuromet) (oxiracetam),
    136–38
neurons, 36, 46–60, 69
    aging and, 50–52
    amino acids and, 152–54, 157–58,
        160, 164–66
    basic components of, 54
    communication between, 53–57,
        64, 73, 139, 160, 167, 179, 216

death of, 35, 50, 64, 82, 107,
131–32, 142, 154, 160, 196,
200, 214–16
and drugs in improving thinking,
64–66
future therapeutic agents and,
213–18
hormones and, 169, 176, 179, 181
information and, 57–60, 64, 82
and negative influences of drugs,
46–49
oxygen and, 206–8, 211
smart drugs and, 73, 75, 79, 82, 85,
87–88, 94–95, 100–101, 107,
122, 125, 127, 131–32, 135,
138–39, 141–42
vitamins and, 192, 196, 200
neuroprotective agents, 214–16
neuroscience, 213
neurosteroids, 179
neurotransmitters, 37, 39, 167
amino acids and, 152–53, 157, 162,
164–65
definition of, 56
and drugs in improving thinking,
64–66
excitatory, see excitatory neurotransmitters
future therapeutic agents and, 215,
219–21
hormones and, 169, 172, 179, 181
information and, 59–60
inhibitory, 57, 59
in neuron communication, 55–57
oxygen and, 203
smart drugs and, 69–75, 79, 84–87,
90, 92, 98, 100–101, 103, 110,
118–19, 125, 127–28, 131,
134–35, 139, 141, 144, 146–47,
149
vitamins and, 188, 190–91
neurotrophic factors, 218–19
niacin (nicotinic acid) (vitamin B₃),
187–90
nimodipine (Nimotop), 130–34
N-methyl-D-aspartate (NMDA)
receptors:
amino acids and, 157–60
future therapeutic agents and, 221

nonsteroidal anti-inflammatory drugs
(NSAIDs), 47–48, 129
nootropics:
definition of, 68
see also smart drugs
Nootropil (piracetam), 74, 86, 136–37,
141–45
norepinephrine, 69, 144
smart drugs and, 87, 103, 146–47

occipital lobe, 59
Olmifon (adrafinil), 69–72
ondansetron (Zofran), 134–36
opium poppies, 26
osteoporosis, 25, 80
Ostfield, A., 103
over-the-counter remedies, 47–49
oxidative stress, 203–4
oxiracetam (Neuroactiv) (Neuromet),
136–38
oxygen, 202–12
oxygen therapies, 204–11

pantothenic acid, 201
parietal lobe, 59
Parkinson's disease:
amino acids and, 159–60
future therapeutic agents and, 215,
217–18
oxygen and, 204
treatment of, 64–66, 89–91, 102–3,
121, 192–93
Parsees, 120–21
Pauling, Linus, 186
Paullinia cupana (guarana), 115–17
pentoxifylline, 220–21
periwinkle plant, 146, 148
phencyclidine (PCP) (Angel Dust),
216
phenytoin (Dilantin), 94–97
phosphatidylcholine, 84–87
phosphatidylserine, 138–41
Physicians' Desk Reference, 97, 121,
133
Physicians' Desk Reference for Herbal
Medicines, 17
physostigmine, 86
piracetam (Nootropil), 74, 86, 136–37,
141–45

placebo-controlled trials, 30–32
  see also double-blind placebo-controlled trials; single-blind placebo-controlled trials
placebo effects, 30–31
placebos:
  animal testing and, 28
  in human testing, 30–32
planning ability, 30
positive mood, 38
Positron Emission Tomographic (PET) scans, 121–22
posture, 37
potassium, 94–95
Practical Guide to Natural Medicines, 17
pramiracetam, 136, 144–45
pregnancy, 17, 25
  hormones and, 172, 174
  vitamins and, 186
pregnenolone, 178–80
prescription drugs, *see* drug, drugs
President's Commission on Dietary Supplement Labels, 15
Princeton University, 221
problem solving, 49
procaine, 102–3
procedural memory, 62–63
progesterone, 92, 178
propentofylline, 220
propranalol hydrochloride (Inderal), 126–30
Prozac, 93
pyridoxine (vitamin B$_6$), 190–93, 201
pyroglutamate, 141, 161–63

Qian Ceng Ta, 117–18

racetams, 74, 136–37, 141, 144
rats:
  amino acids and, 162
  future therapeutic agents and, 219–20
  genetics and, 46
  hormones and, 176, 179
  oxygen and, 209–10
  smart drugs and, 70, 72–73, 75, 78, 82, 88, 91, 93, 110, 112, 119–20, 132, 139, 142, 144, 146–47

testing drugs and dietary supplements on, 29
reaction times:
  smart drugs and, 111
  vitamins and, 194
reasoning ability, 61
recreational drugs, 49–50, 69, 195
retention, 51
retirement, 52
riboflavin (vitamin B$_2$), 191, 201
risk/benefit ratios:
  amino acids and, 163
  of drugs, 21–35
  of herbal remedies, 11–15
  hormones and, 180
  smart drugs and, 96, 114, 130
Ritalin, 64
rolziracetam, 136, 144

St. John's Wort, 11–12, 14
sedatives, 33
seizures, *see* epilepsy
selegiline hydrochloride (deprenyl) (Eldepryl), 89–93
semantic memory, 62–63
senility:
  amino acids and, 161
  genetics and, 45
  oxygen and, 208
  smart drugs and, 77, 83, 100–101, 110, 119, 121, 124, 137, 140, 142, 145, 150
  and testing drugs and dietary supplements, 35
  vitamins and, 190
serotonin, 103, 134–35, 144
serotonin-reuptake inhibitors, 93
short-term memory, 62–63
  amino acids and, 165
  oxygen and, 210
  smart drugs and, 107, 142, 150
  vitamins and, 188–89
Siberian ginseng, 109, 111
single-blind placebo-controlled trials, 31–32, 133
  smart drugs and, 80, 110
skin, skin disorders, 33, 42, 96
sleep, sleep problems, 33, 37
  hormones and, 179

smart drugs and, 69, 71, 80, 92, 96,
    101, 109, 111, 115, 117, 123,
    129, 146–47
smart drugs, 68–151
    amino acids and, 75, 118–19, 125,
        131, 139, 141, 157, 159
    definition of, 68
    hormones and, 167, 175–76, 178
    interactions of, 71, 92–93, 96–97,
        128–29, 133
    research and, 214
    side effects of, 71–74, 79–80, 82,
        86, 88–89, 91–94, 96–97,
        101–2, 107–8, 111, 113–14,
        116, 119, 123, 125, 128–29,
        133, 135–38, 141–42, 145, 150
    vitamins and, 193, 199
Smart Drugs (Dean and
    Morganthaler), 127n, 133
social comprehension, 95
Society for Neuroscience, 213
sodium, 94–95, 149
somas (dendrites), 54–56
somatotropin (somatotrophic hor-
    mone) (growth hormone),
    175–78
spatial memory, 206
speech problems, see verbal fluency
stress, 40, 65, 69
    aging and, 51–52
    impact on brain of, 37–38
    and negative influences of drugs,
        47–48
    oxygen and, 212
    smart drugs and, 109, 127–30, 140
striatum, 59, 61
stroke, 33
    future therapeutic agents and,
        217–18, 220
    hormones and, 175
    oxygen and, 210
    smart drugs and, 88, 132–34, 146,
        148–49
surgery, 14, 61
synapses, 54–56, 167
    amino acids and, 157
    future therapeutic agents and,
        215
    information and, 59–60

smart drugs and, 82, 100–101,
    118–19, 139
synaptic vesicles, 56
Syntopressin (Diapid) (vasopressin)
    (antidiuretic hormone) (ADH)
    (Ditressin), 180–84
talepetrako (Hydrocotyle asiatica)
    (Indian pennywort) (Centella
    asiatica) (gotu kola), 112–14
Tap (idebenone) (Avan), 124–26
taurine, 164–66
temporal lobe, 59, 61–62
testing:
    amino acids and, 154–55, 158–59,
        162, 165
    on animals, see animal testing
    of dietary supplements, 23–24,
        26–32, 34–35
    future therapeutic agents and,
        217–21
    hormones and, 170, 173–74, 176,
        179, 181–84
    on humans, see human testing
    oxygen and, 206, 209–10
    smart drugs and, 72–73, 75–76, 78,
        80–83, 85–86, 88, 90–91, 93,
        95, 98–104, 106–8, 110–11,
        113–16, 119–20, 122–23, 125,
        128, 132–33, 135, 137, 139–40,
        142–49
    vitamins and, 188–89, 191, 194–95,
        197, 199–200
    see also double-blind placebo-
        controlled trials; single-blind
        placebo-controlled trials
testosterone, 39, 168–69, 171
thiamine (vitamin B₁), 186, 193–95
thinking abilities:
    aging and, 51
    drugs in improvement of, 64–67
    moods and, 37
    MSG and, 42–43
    and negative influences of drugs, 47
    smart drugs and, 68
    and testing drugs and dietary sup-
        plements, 27–28
    see also specific thinking abilities
thyroid hormones, 38–40, 167
tranquilizers, 33, 47, 142

tricyclic antidepressants, 93
triglycerides, 218
tyramine, 93

Valium, 47
vasopressin (antidiuretic hormone)
    (ADH) (Ditressin)
    (Syntopressin) (Diapid), 180–84
verapamil, 133
verbal fluency, 11–12
    aging and, 51
    amino acids and, 154–55
    animal testing and, 29
    hormones and, 39, 173–76
    smart drugs and, 132
verbal memory, 63
    amino acids and, 162
    smart drugs and, 88, 107
vigilance, 206
vincamine, 145–48
vinpocetine (Cavinton), 148–51
Visilor (fipexide) (Attentil) (BP662),
    100–102
visual memory, 63, 107, 132
visuomotor coordination, 95
visuospatial perceptual functions, 51
vitamins, 25, 68, 96, 186–201
    A, 199
    B, 25, 186–98, 201

B_1 (thiamine), 186, 193–95
B_2 (riboflavin), 191, 201
B_3 (niacin), 187–90
B_6 (pyridoxine), 190–93, 201
B_{12} (cyanocobalamin), 196–98
C, 186, 199, 201
    definition of, 186
E (alpha-tocopherol), 199–201
    interactions of, 189
    side effects of, 189

warfarin (Coumadin), 33, 107–8, 111,
    117, 140, 150
water, hyper-oxygenated, 212
water hyssop (bacopa) (brahmi), 77–79
weakness, 42
white blood cell counts, 88–89
Wisniewski, Henry, 43
working memory, 62–63

xanthine derivatives, 220–21
xanthinol nicotinate, 188–89

Yale Mental Health Clinical Research
    Center, 30–31
yohimbine, 71
Yokon, 71

Zofran (ondansetron), 134–36

THEODORE I. LIDSKY, Ph.D., is a neuroscientist who specializes in research on the brain and behavior with a particular interest in the effects of environmental neurotoxins on the developing brain. He maintains an active research laboratory supported by governmental and private funding and has published numerous papers in peer-reviewed scientific/medical journals concerning brain function and behavior.

Dr. Lidsky holds a B.A. in psychology from Queens College of the City University of New York and a Ph.D. from the University of Rochester. He received postdoctoral training at the Mental Retardation Center of the Neuropsychiatric Institute at the University of California at Los Angeles.

His professional experience began in 1975 at the State University of New York at Stony Brook, where he served as a tenured faculty member in the Psychology Department performing research on the brain and behavior and teaching classes on psychology, neuropsychology, and neuroscience to undergraduate, graduate, and medical students. He moved to the Virginia Polytechnic Institute in 1983, where he taught neuroscience in the College of Veterinary Medicine. In 1986, Dr. Lidsky joined the faculty of the Sophie Davis School of Biomedical Education, where he taught physiology, pharmacology, and neuroscience.

He assumed his current position in 1989 at the New York

State Institute for Basic Research in Developmental Disabilities, where he directs the Laboratory of Electrophysiology. In addition, Dr. Lidsky is an adjunct associate professor of neurology at Thomas Jefferson University Medical School, where with coauthor Dr. Jay Schneider, he directs the Neurofunctional Assessment Unit.

JAY S. SCHNEIDER, Ph.D., has authored more than 100 papers in the field of neuroscience, including numerous papers dealing with drug effects on the brain and behavior. His research runs the gamut from molecular biology to human clinical drug studies. Dr. Schneider specializes in the study of Parkinson's disease and maintains active research programs in the fields of neurodegeneration, neurotoxicology, and behavioral pharmacology. He also has presented over 120 papers and talks at international scientific meetings. In addition to the two books Dr. Schneider coauthored with Dr. Lidsky, he has edited *Current Concepts in Parkinson's Disease Research* and *Sphingolipids in Health and Medicine* for the professional community, and has contributed numerous chapters to other books.

Dr. Schneider holds a B.A. in psychology from the State University of New York at Stony Brook, where he also received his Ph.D. He served as a postdoctoral research fellow in the Department of Psychiatry and in the Neuropsychiatric Institute at the University of California, Los Angeles (UCLA). He became an assistant professor of neurology at UCLA in 1983; moved to Hahnemann University, where he served as an associate professor of neurology until 1997; and currently serves as professor of pathology, anatomy, and cell biology and professor of neurology at Thomas Jefferson University in Philadelphia, where he also directs the Parkinson's Disease Research Unit and codirects the Neurofunctional Assessment Unit with Dr. Lidsky.

9 780684 870809